WORD SEARCH
BIBLE PUZZLE BOOK

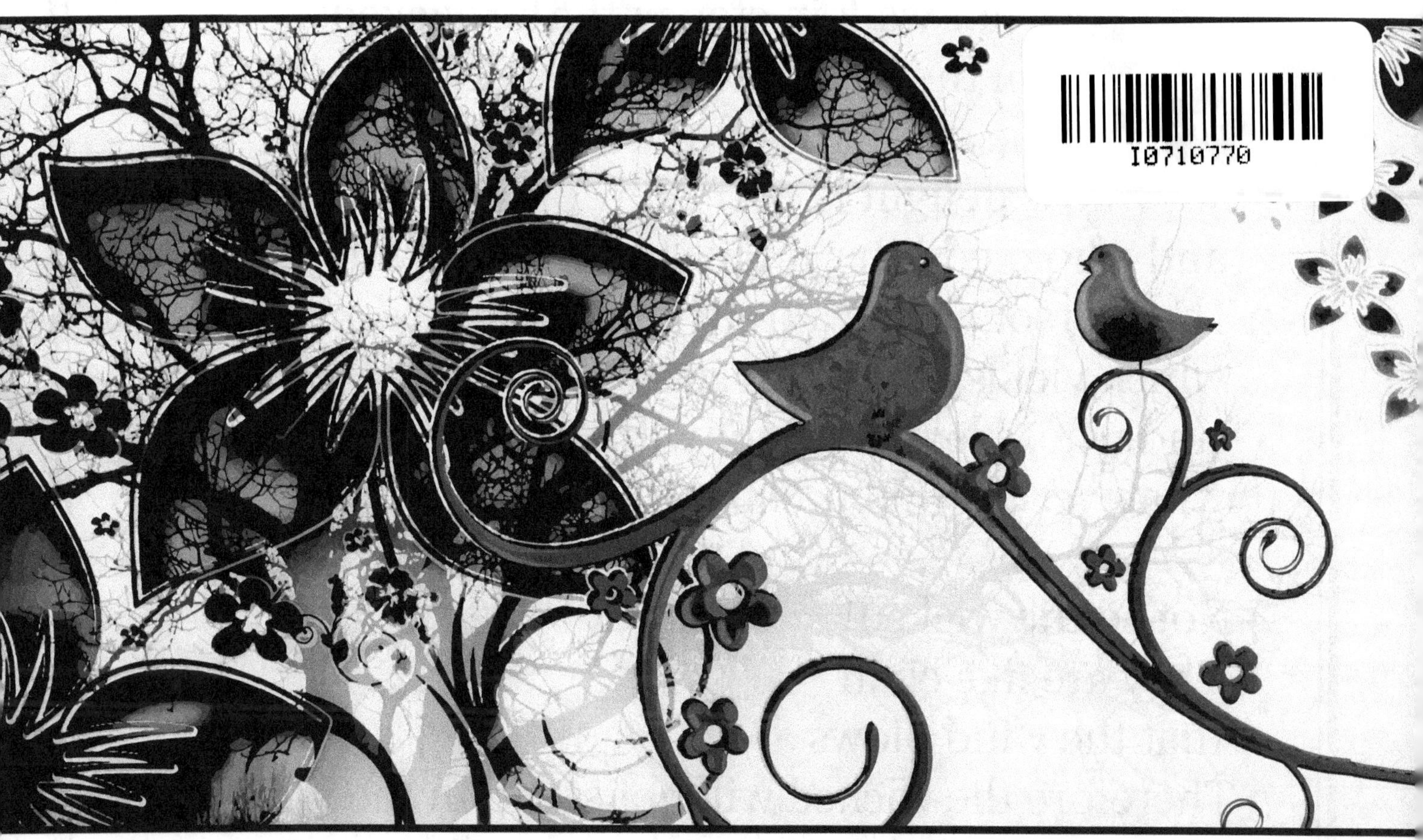

PSALMS & HYMNS

Wth Text · Large Print

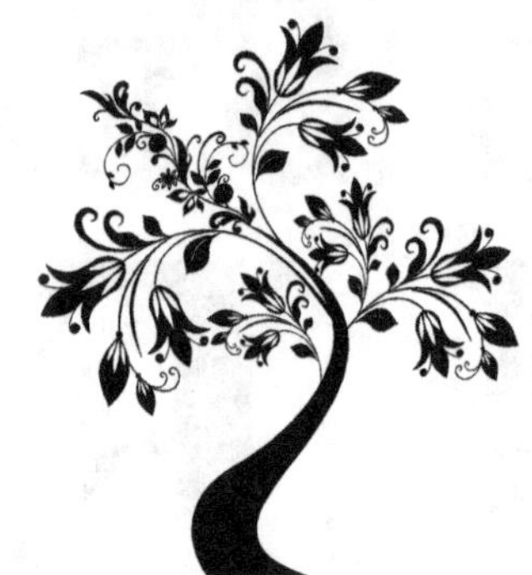

1 Blessed is the one
   who does not walk in step with the wicked
    or stand in the way that sinners take
    or sit in the company of mockers,
2 but whose delight is in the law of the LORD,
    and who meditates on his law day and night.
3 That person is like a tree planted by streams of water,
    which yields its fruit in season
    and whose leaf does not wither—
    whatever they do prospers.

4 Not so the wicked!
    They are like chaff
    that the wind blows away.
5 Therefore the wicked will not stand in the judgment,
    nor sinners in the assembly of the righteous.

6 For the LORD watches over the way of the righteous,
    but the way of the wicked leads to destruction

Psalm 1

Psalm 1

```
B P T N O H Z K L A W V
A R P F R T P M G B I T
N O P F I G C A K L N T
C S D R G J S S N E D V
O P X U H M A S M S W K
M E D I T A T E S S A R
P R B T E D G M G E T Q
A S M F O D C B H D C H
N T O C U D E L I G H T
Y J B J S W A Y I Y E R
S O B E J Y I E L D S E
E O E T J B F M L Y N E
```

BLESSED	TREE	JUDGEMENT
COMPANY	YIELDS	ASSEMBLY
DELIGHT	FRUIT	RIGHTEOUS
LAW	PROSPERS	WATCHES
MEDITATES	WIND	WAY

Answer on Page 102

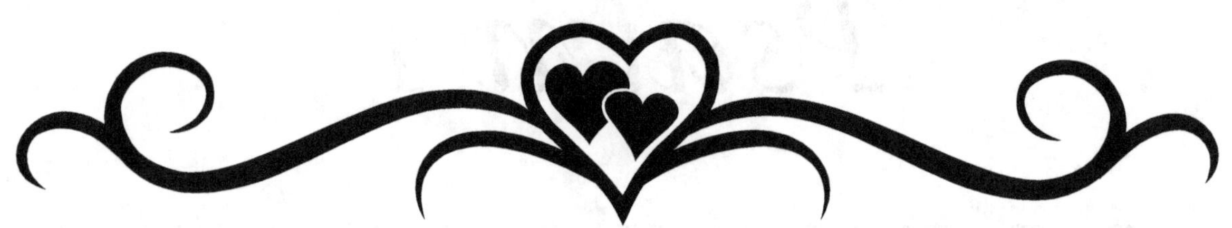

5 Offer the sacrifices of the righteous
    and trust in the LORD.

6 Many, LORD, are asking, "Who will bring us
    prosperity?"
    Let the light of your face shine on us.
7 Fill my heart with joy
    when their grain and new wine abound.

8 In peace I will lie down and sleep,
    for you alone, LORD,
    make me dwell in safety.

Psalm 4:5-8

Psalm 4:5-8

```
D X H E D V D Y D N S J
P I F N Z P V J J O Y J
W Y K A G T R U S T X Q
V I S A C R I F I C E S
W E N Y H E A R T V A M
S A P E A C E I X T F C
A O K C U P T Z N U F O
F S C S S H I N E P U N
E Y K O G D M L B C G Z
T G R I G H T E O U S E
Y P L U N D W E L L I S
V F M C J G C M L Y O F
```

SACRIFICES	WINE	HEART
LIGHT	TRUST	DWELL
GRAIN	SHINE	PROSPERITY
RIGHTEOUS	PEACE	JOY
FACE	ASKING	SAFETY

Answer on Page 102

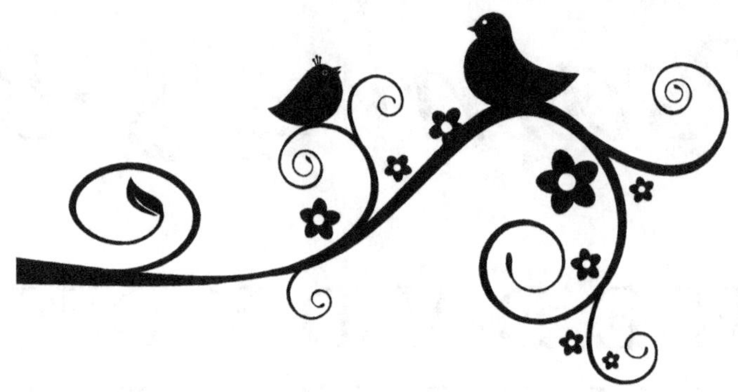

5 You have made them a little lower than the
    angels
  and crowned them with glory and honor.
6 You made them rulers over the works of
    your hands;
  you put everything under their feet:
7 all flocks and herds,
    and the animals of the wild,
8 the birds in the sky,
    and the fish in the sea,
    all that swim the paths of the seas.

9 LORD, our LORD,
    how majestic is your name in all the earth!

Psalm 8:5-9

Psalm 8:5-9

H	A	N	D	S	K	Y	C	R	W	Y	V
H	N	N	P	S	N	U	Y	A	G	L	N
V	I	Y	G	C	R	O	W	N	E	D	C
T	M	A	J	E	S	T	I	C	J	U	B
S	A	L	G	L	L	H	E	R	D	S	F
A	L	R	L	V	T	S	O	Y	W	A	E
Y	S	U	O	Y	Z	T	S	N	X	B	A
Z	Q	L	R	E	Q	K	I	T	O	I	R
K	G	E	Y	T	C	W	T	F	Q	R	T
W	V	R	W	O	L	F	S	O	I	D	H
E	Y	S	L	F	C	F	F	X	D	S	C
Z	E	F	D	S	B	E	K	F	U	T	H

ANGELS	HANDS	BIRDS
CROWNED	EVERYTHING	SKY
GLORY	FLOCKS	FISH
HONOR	HERDS	MAJESTIC
RULERS	ANIMALS	EARTH

Answer on Page 102

1 How long, LORD? Will you forget me forever?
  How long will you hide your face from me?
2 How long must I wrestle with my thoughts
  and day after day have sorrow in my heart?
  How long will my enemy triumph over me?

3 Look on me and answer, LORD my GOD.
  Give light to my eyes, or I will sleep in death,
4 and my enemy will say, "I have overcome him,"
  and my foes will rejoice when I fall.

5 But I trust in your unfailing love;
  my heart rejoices in your salvation.
6 I will sing the LORD's praise,
  for he has been good to me.

Psalm 13

Psalm 13

J	M	C	R	F	V	D	F	D	R	S	V
K	J	K	T	H	O	U	G	H	T	S	Z
P	H	A	Z	O	L	N	F	T	I	W	X
R	R	N	G	X	O	F	R	R	S	D	K
A	Q	S	A	L	V	A	T	I	O	N	E
B	J	W	N	Y	E	I	U	U	R	R	C
A	L	E	H	H	R	L	X	M	R	E	S
K	O	R	N	I	C	I	Z	P	O	J	Y
U	Y	O	B	L	O	N	G	H	W	O	X
V	X	X	O	R	M	G	U	Z	R	I	L
C	C	A	W	R	E	S	T	L	E	C	A
W	C	A	K	M	X	E	F	A	C	E	Y

LONG   SORROW   REJOICE

HIDE   HEART   UNFAILING

FACE   TRIUMPH   LOVE

WRESTLE   ANSWER   SALVATION

THOUGHTS   OVERCOME   GOOD

Answer on Page 102

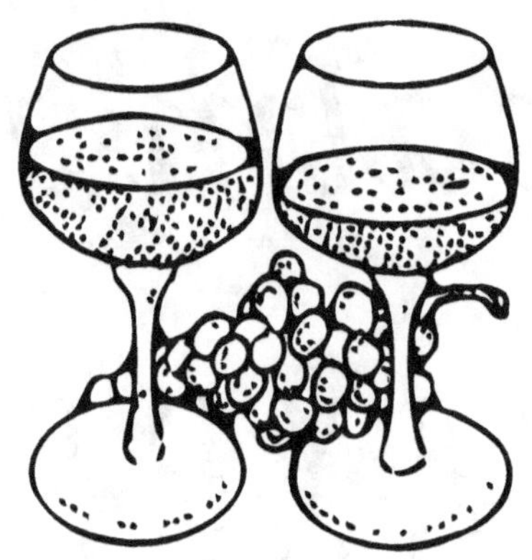

5 LORD, you alone are my portion and my cup;
　you make my lot secure.
6 The boundary lines have fallen for me in pleasant
　　places; surely I have a delightful inheritance.
7 I will praise the LORD, who counsels me;
　even at night my heart instructs me.
8 I keep my eyes always on the LORD.
　With him at my right hand, I will not be shaken.

9　Therefore my heart is glad and my tongue rejoices;
　　my body also will rest secure,
10 because you will not abandon me to the realm of
　　the dead,
　　nor will you let your faithful one see decay.
11 You make known to me the path of life;
　you will fill me with joy in your presence,
　with eternal pleasures at your right hand.

Psalm 16:5-8

Psalm 16:5-8

M	X	Z	M	F	K	Y	J	F	B	U	R
D	B	Y	V	P	S	E	C	U	R	E	I
H	R	O	M	E	L	H	Z	I	C	Y	S
W	F	E	U	I	T	E	A	N	Q	L	B
T	P	A	E	N	I	E	A	K	E	Q	L
X	O	E	I	S	D	T	R	S	E	K	W
S	R	N	Q	T	I	A	N	N	A	N	H
S	T	B	G	R	H	U	R	O	A	N	V
X	I	H	E	U	O	F	C	Y	Z	L	T
V	O	H	C	C	E	J	U	F	T	V	G
E	N	P	A	T	H	W	P	L	E	I	M
I	P	R	E	S	E	N	C	E	Y	E	S

PORTION
CUP
SECURE
BOUNDARY
PLEASANT
INHERITANCE
COUNSELS
INSTRUCTS
EYES
SHAKEN
TONGUE
FAITHFUL
PATH
PRESENCE
ETERNAL

Answer on Page 103

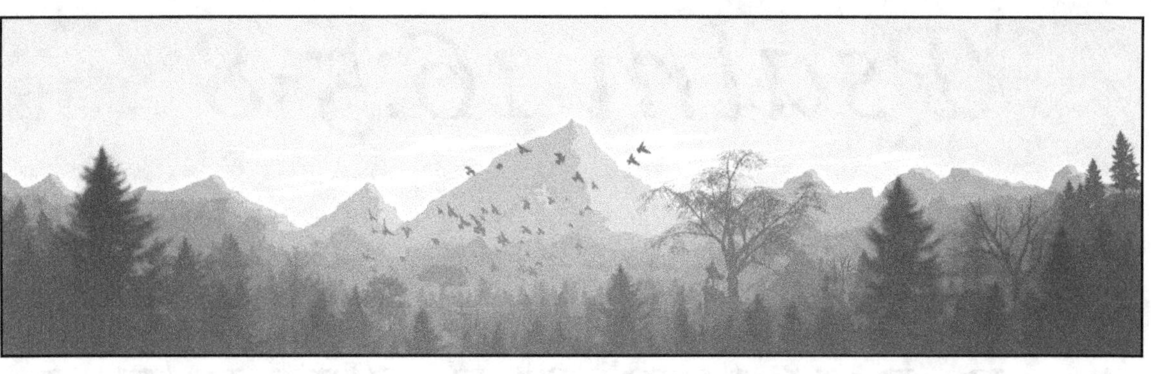

1 I love you, LORD, my strength.

2 The LORD is my rock, my fortress and my
    deliverer;
  my GOD is my rock, in whom I take refuge,
  my shield and the horn of my salvation, my
    strong hold.

3 I called to the LORD, who is worthy of praise,
    and I have been saved from my enemies.
4 The cords of death entangled me;
    the torrents of destruction overwhelmed me.
5 The cords of the grave coiled around me;
    the snares of death confronted me.

Psalm 18:1-5

Psalm 18:1-5

U	O	V	E	R	W	H	E	L	M	E	D
E	N	T	A	N	G	L	E	D	D	S	E
S	N	A	R	E	S	A	Z	S	Y	T	L
S	A	L	V	A	T	I	O	N	W	R	I
X	Z	S	H	I	E	L	D	Y	R	O	V
D	E	S	T	R	U	C	T	I	O	N	E
F	O	R	T	R	E	S	S	P	C	G	R
P	O	J	I	W	E	F	D	B	K	H	E
D	G	B	B	N	J	N	U	T	E	O	R
B	Y	S	R	G	F	H	G	G	C	L	L
K	C	O	N	F	R	O	N	T	E	D	B
F	H	I	A	E	W	O	R	T	H	Y	H

STRENGTH   SHIELD   ENTANGLED
ROCK   HORN   DESTRUCTION
FORTRESS   SALVATION   CONFRONTED
DELIVERER   STRONG HOLD   SNARES
REFUGE   WORTHY   OVERWHELMED

Answer on Page 103

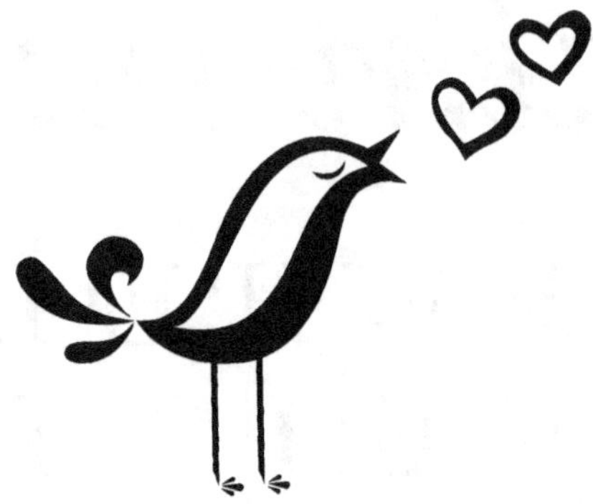

1 The heavens declare the glory of GOD;
  the skies proclaim the work of his hands.
2 Day after day they pour forth speech;
  night after night they reveal knowledge.
3 They have no speech, they use no words;
  no sound is heard from them.
4 Yet their voice goes out into all the earth,
  their words to the ends of the world.
  In the heavens GOD has pitched a tent
    for the sun.
5 It is like a bridegroom coming out of his chamber,
  like a champion rejoicing to run his course.
6 It rises at one end of the heavens
  and makes its circuit to the other;
  nothing is deprived of its warmth.

Psalm 19:1-6

Psalm 19:1-6

H	V	S	K	F	S	H	W	O	R	L	D
W	O	P	N	A	V	Q	X	W	A	A	G
O	I	E	O	H	F	H	T	E	N	T	W
R	C	E	W	E	E	S	V	F	C	N	Z
D	E	C	L	A	R	E	P	G	H	K	U
S	I	H	E	V	R	N	R	L	A	J	W
B	R	I	D	E	G	R	O	O	M	K	O
U	H	W	G	N	W	O	C	R	P	D	P
S	K	I	E	S	Y	D	L	Y	I	M	O
B	K	O	J	S	V	F	A	Y	O	Q	K
O	P	W	K	Z	J	U	I	Y	N	V	K
U	D	I	R	W	A	R	M	T	H	T	L

HEAVENS	SPEECH	WORLD
DECLARE	REVEAL	TENT
GLORY	KNOWLEDGE	BRIDEGROOM
SKIES	VOICE	CHAMPION
PROCLAIM	WORDS	WARMTH

Answer on Page 103

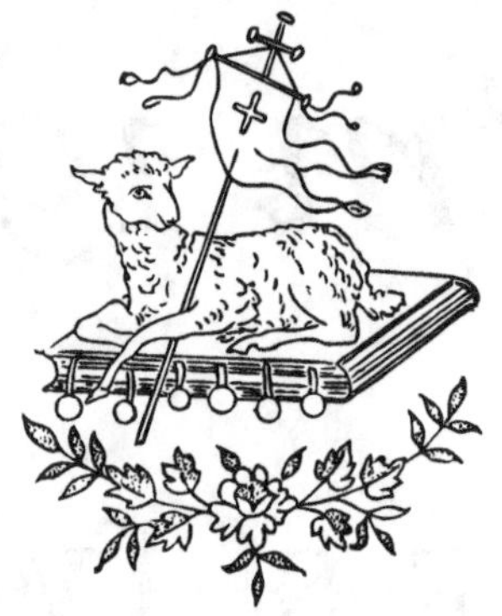

1 The LORD is my shepherd, I lack nothing.
2 He makes me lie down in green pastures,
    he leads me beside quiet waters,
3 he refreshes my soul.
    He guides me along the right paths
    for his name's sake.
4 Even though I walk
    through the darkest valley, I will fear no evil,
    for you are with me; your rod and your staff,
    they comfort me.

5 You prepare a table before me
    in the presence of my enemies.
    You anoint my head with oil;
    my cup overflows.
6 Surely your goodness and love will follow me
    all the days of my life,
    and I will dwell in the house of the LORD forever.

Psalm 23

Psalm 23

Q	A	K	S	A	A	Z	T	C	V	Q	M
W	P	S	R	O	D	X	E	R	V	X	L
L	A	R	H	G	U	I	D	E	S	O	J
Y	B	T	E	E	O	L	J	S	H	C	N
C	D	F	E	P	P	O	E	W	Q	B	O
S	O	N	N	R	A	H	D	P	S	N	K
L	V	M	V	O	S	R	E	N	K	A	J
H	A	G	F	E	T	S	E	R	E	S	D
F	L	C	R	O	U	H	T	F	D	S	Q
Q	L	F	K	W	R	Z	I	A	O	X	S
I	E	X	B	Y	E	T	E	N	F	C	G
R	Y	W	U	J	S	L	L	N	G	F	X

SHEPHERD	WATERS	ROD
LACK	REFRESHES	STAFF
NOTHING	SOUL	COMFORT
PASTURES	GUIDES	PREPARE
LEADS	VALLEY	GOODNESS

Answer on Page 103

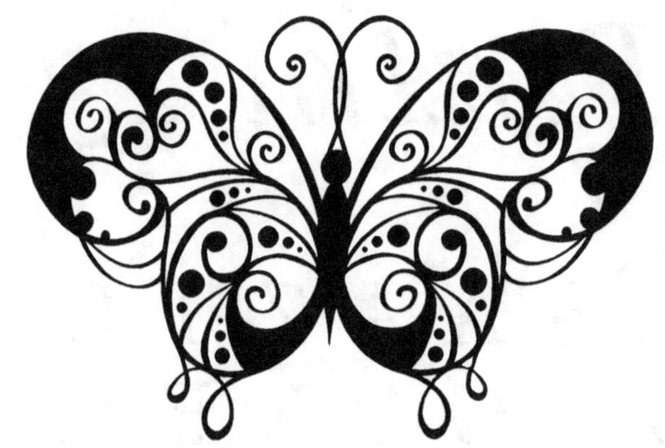

1 The earth is the LORD's, and everything in it,
   the world, and all who live in it;
2 for he founded it on the seas
   and established it on the waters.

3 Who may ascend the mountain of the LORD?
   Who may stand in his holy place?
4 The one who has clean hands and a pure heart,
   who does not trust in an idol
   or swear by a false god.

5 They will receive blessing from the LORD
   and vindication from GOD their Savior.
6 Such is the generation of those who seek him,
   who seek your face, GOD of Jacob.

Psalm 24:1-6

Psalm 24:1-6

P	X	C	E	K	E	V	Q	X	P	D	H
U	B	L	E	S	S	I	N	G	E	P	X
R	A	E	M	T	E	N	N	H	U	N	U
E	S	A	O	A	A	D	S	K	O	X	E
K	A	N	U	N	S	I	D	I	C	L	K
B	S	R	N	D	L	C	T	H	R	Z	Y
V	C	I	T	B	O	A	E	M	D	A	J
I	F	C	A	H	R	T	H	N	W	J	Y
T	M	T	I	E	D	I	L	Q	D	G	Y
N	S	L	N	I	S	O	P	V	V	H	E
E	M	E	F	O	U	N	D	E	D	I	B
R	G	Q	O	W	R	Z	E	Y	D	N	U

EARTH	ASCEND	PURE
LORD	MOUNTAIN	BLESSING
FOUNDED	STAND	VINDICATION
SEAS	HOLY	GENERATION
ESTABLISHED	CLEAN	SEEK

Answer on Page 104

1 In you, LORD my GOD,
   I put my trust.

2 I trust in you;
   do not let me be put to shame,
   nor let my enemies triumph over me.
3 No one who hopes in you
   will ever be put to shame,
   but shame will come on those
   who are treacherous without cause.

4 Show me your ways, LORD,
   teach me your paths.
5 Guide me in your truth and teach me,
   for you are GOD my Savior,
   and my hope is in you all day long.
6 Remember, LORD, your great mercy and love,
   for they are from of old.

Psalm 25:1-6

Psalm 25:1-6

Q	Q	O	P	M	E	O	S	V	S	S	W
D	J	T	R	U	T	H	E	S	D	S	E
E	Y	E	B	W	T	P	Q	X	U	A	T
X	P	J	G	A	A	T	M	O	V	V	Y
B	G	N	P	U	E	Y	R	W	A	I	Y
L	E	N	E	M	I	E	S	U	X	O	S
G	T	E	A	C	H	O	P	E	S	R	F
V	U	H	W	C	O	C	Y	Q	H	T	V
G	S	I	A	P	Z	C	J	G	O	P	H
Z	O	E	D	W	R	J	U	J	W	G	Y
R	R	E	M	E	M	B	E	R	V	S	O
T	X	S	M	B	X	L	G	S	H	U	U

PUT TRUST
SHAME
ENEMIES
HOPES
TREACHEROUS
SHOW
WAYS
TEACH
PATHS
GUIDE
TRUTH
SAVIOR
DAY
REMEMBER
MERCY

Answer on Page 104

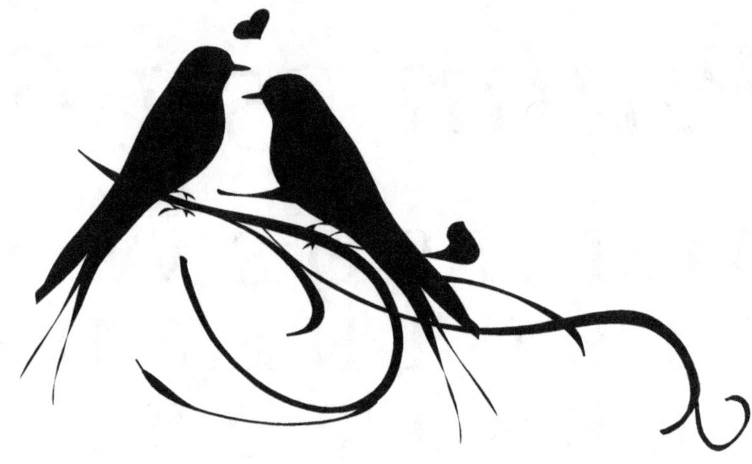

1 I will exalt you, LORD,
   for you lifted me out of the depths
   and did not let my enemies gloat over me.
2 Lord my GOD, I called to you for help,
   and you healed me.
3 You, LORD, brought me up from the realm of the dead;
   you spared me from going down to the pit.

4 Sing the praises of the LORD, you his faithful people;
   praise his holy name.
5 For his anger lasts only a moment,
   but his favor lasts a lifetime;
   weeping may stay for the night,
   but rejoicing comes in the morning

Psalm 30:1-5

Psalm 30:1-5

O	F	P	X	B	M	K	J	M	M	C	R
X	K	M	G	L	O	A	T	F	Y	U	O
H	H	P	O	B	M	W	W	P	E	M	U
X	E	N	D	R	E	W	X	N	K	S	D
C	L	H	C	O	N	G	O	T	U	P	D
E	P	V	A	U	T	I	M	A	F	A	T
X	R	L	L	G	B	B	N	H	I	R	D
A	A	I	L	H	T	R	G	G	E	E	I
L	I	F	E	T	I	M	E	M	L	D	T
T	S	T	D	E	L	G	I	A	H	D	V
W	E	E	P	I	N	G	E	U	L	I	Z
D	S	D	E	P	T	H	S	O	P	M	W

EXALT	HELP	PRAISES
LIFTED	HEALED	MOMENT
DEPTHS	BROUGHT	LIFETIME
GLOAT	REALM	WEEPING
CALLED	SPARED	MORNING

Answer on Page 104

1 I will extol the LORD at all times;
  his praise will always be on my lips.
2 I will glory in the LORD;
  let the afflicted hear and rejoice.
3 Glorify the LORD with me;
  let us exalt his name together.

4 I sought the LORD, and he answered me;
  he delivered me from all my fears.
5 Those who look to him are radiant;
  their faces are never covered with shame.
6 This poor man called, and the LORD heard him;
  he saved him out of all his troubles.
7 The angel of the LORD encamps around those
  who fear him, and he delivers them.

Psalm 34:1-7

Psalm 34:1-7

```
A V O Q F V T A Y F J Q
N T R J G U O F A C E S
S R E Z E D G F J O D L
W O A G E E E L S X A A
E U N L C L T I A U O J
R B G O P I H C V S U N
E L E R J V E T E L S E
D E L I V E R E D E L X
Z S I F N R A D I A N T
D R P Y A S O U G H T O
Y M S E N D N T O B W L
B H H T C K Y Y Y H P S
```

EXTOL	TOGETHER	FACES
LIPS	SOUGHT	SAVED
AFFLICTED	ANSWERED	TROUBLES
HEAR	DELIVERED	ANGEL
GLORIFY	RADIANT	DELIVERS

Answer on Page 104

3 Trust in the LORD and do good;
  dwell in the land and enjoy safe pasture.
4 Take delight in the LORD,
  and he will give you the desires of your heart.

5 Commit your way to the LORD;
  trust in him and he will do this:
6 He will make your righteous reward shine like the
  dawn, your vindication like the noonday sun.

7 Be still before the LORD
  and wait patiently for him;
  do not fret when people succeed in their ways,
  when they carry out their wicked schemes.

8 Refrain from anger and turn from wrath;
  do not fret—it leads only to evil.
9 For those who are evil will be destroyed,
  but those who hope in the LORD will inherit the land.

Psalm 37:3-9

Psalm 37:3-9

X F L V O Z Y S Q Y R T
W V A G P K U J V L E S
B I N D A W N I L U W R
F N D E S I R E S O A C
V D B M T W W T F S R S
M I P I U D O G O O D O
P C A R R Y E N J O Y C
P A T I E N T L Y A E O
N T V C I V F X I E A M
R I I H K N B Q C G F M
N O S U C C E E D F H I
R N L Y Y F T N W B B T

DO GOOD	DELIGHT	DAWN
DWELL	DESIRES	VINDICATION
LAND	COMMIT	PATIENTLY
ENJOY	REWARD	SUCCEED
PASTURE	SHINE	CARRY

Answer on Page 105

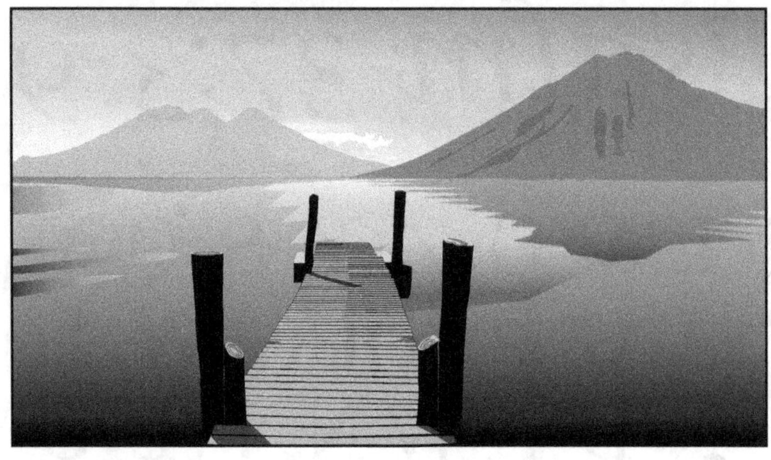

1 GOD is our refuge and strength,
   an ever-present help in trouble.
2 Therefore we will not fear, though the earth
   give way and the mountains fall into the
   heart of the sea,
3 though its waters roar and foam
   and the mountains quake with their surging.

4 There is a river whose streams make glad the
   city of GOD, the holy place where the
   Most High dwells.
5 GOD is within her, she will not fall;
   GOD will help her at break of day.
6 Nations are in uproar, kingdoms fall;
   he lifts his voice, the earth melts.

Psalm 46:1-6

Psalm 46:1-6

```
M O S T H I G H C I T Y
U H K T W I T H I N R P
O J L I R G G R E O I B
S T U W N E L K O X V N
W U P E J G A H C A E U
M B R E L U D M T M R Q
D T O G Q Y A O S T Q T
S N A T I O N S M B Z N
J P R D F N U C R S W W
P V R E F U G E L M E S
Q Z G R F T M T L Q T F
G M I H C T W F O B Z M
```

REFUGE   SURGING   MOST HIGH
STRENGTH   RIVER   WITHIN
ROAR   STREAMS   NATIONS
FOAM   GLAD   UPROAR
QUAKE   CITY   KINGDOMS

10 Create in me a pure heart, O GOD,
    and renew a steadfast spirit within me.
11 Do not cast me from your presence
    or take your Holy Spirit from me.
12 Restore to me the joy of your salvation
    and grant me a willing spirit, to sustain me.

13 Then I will teach transgressors your ways,
    so that sinners will turn back to you.
14 Deliver me from the guilt of bloodshed, O GOD,
    you who are GOD my Savior,
    and my tongue will sing of your righteousness.
15 Open my lips, LORD,
    and my mouth will declare your praise.

Psalm 51:10-15

Psalm 51:10-15

I	S	U	H	V	A	C	J	U	O	E	N	F
T	V	T	Q	H	D	G	Z	S	S	X	U	R
E	D	C	E	E	K	V	U	K	B	H	T	K
D	E	C	R	A	W	F	F	I	E	Q	B	T
U	C	Q	Y	E	D	W	I	L	L	I	N	G
N	L	T	N	O	A	F	O	I	S	T	N	E
X	A	E	R	Q	P	T	A	P	U	I	R	M
T	R	A	N	S	G	R	E	S	S	O	R	S
U	E	C	N	L	F	S	R	R	T	N	B	T
R	W	H	W	P	D	B	Z	S	A	K	H	F
N	A	K	Y	U	U	B	E	Y	I	K	P	P
H	I	F	S	P	I	R	I	T	N	Y	W	S
L	E	M	D	V	B	G	E	O	X	F	R	B

CREATE	RESTORE	TURN
PURE	WILLING	GUILT
RENEW	SUSTAIN	SING
STEADFAST	TEACH	LIPS
SPIRIT	TRANSGRESSORS	DECLARE

Answer on Page 105

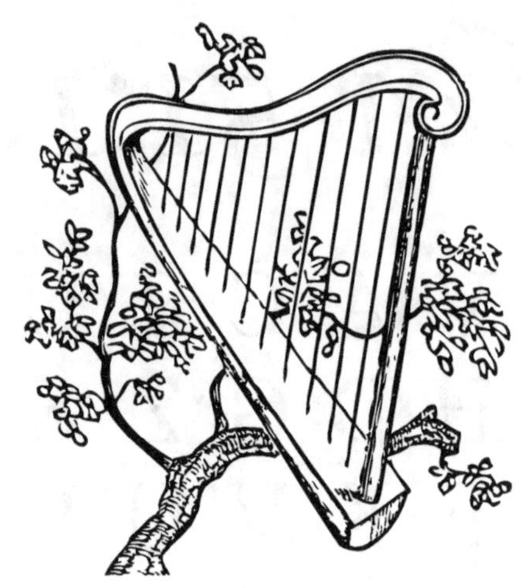

7   My heart, O GOD, is steadfast,
      my heart is steadfast;
      I will sing and make music.
8 Awake, my soul!
      Awake, harp and lyre!
      I will awaken the dawn.

9   I will praise you, LORD, among the nations;
      I will sing of you among the peoples.
10 For great is your love, reaching to the heavens;
      your faithfulness reaches to the skies.

11 Be exalted, O GOD, above the heavens;
      let your glory be over all the earth.

Psalm 57:7-11

Psalm 57:7-11

```
Z Z O A K Y R G L O R Y
Q N G D A W N M U S I C
X K A D H I J G E T Q Y
F A I T H F U L N E S S
J U V C I S P Y W A I K
O H A R P O W R V D H E
A E D B E U N E L F K M
R A C P O L K S A A E V
Y V W N H V V Z W S K E
I E S M Y H E A R T X I
B N R G X B Q N A N U A
Q S G M T S N Z N N V B
```

MY HEART	HARP	REACHING
STEADFAST	LYRE	HEAVENS
MUSIC	DAWN	FAITHFULNESS
AWAKE	NATIONS	ABOVE
SOUL	PEOPLES	GLORY

Answer on Page 105

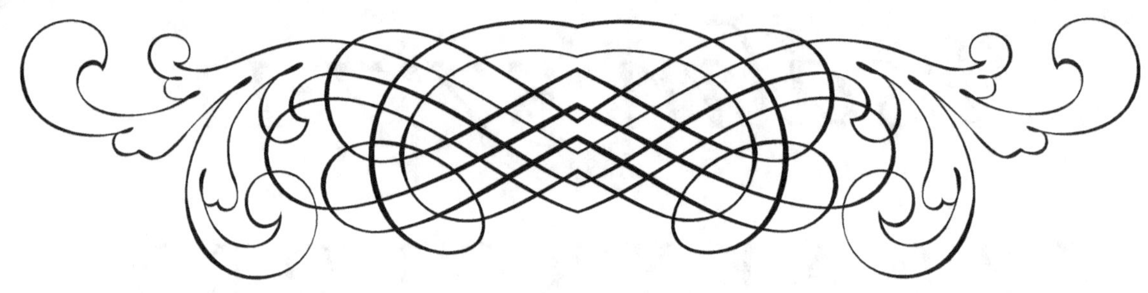

1 Shout for joy to GOD, all the earth!
2 Sing the glory of his name;
     make his praise glorious.
3 Say to GOD, "How awesome are your deeds!
     So great is your power
     that your enemies cringe before you.
4 All the earth bows down to you;
     they sing praise to you,
     they sing the praises of your name."

5 Come and see what GOD has done,
     his awesome deeds for mankind!
6 He turned the sea into dry land,
     they passed through the waters on foot—
     come, let us rejoice in him.
7 He rules forever by his power,
     his eyes watch the nations—
     let not the rebellious rise up against him.

Psalm 66:1-7

Psalm 66:1-7

```
R P E R U J N D K W A G
V W M F O R E V E R W B
K A P A W E S O M E B O
A T U R N E D C G B D W
P C H F L K Q N I E Z S
A H R U B M I R A L S P
Z I R R F S B N L L H A
R P X P R P D K D I O S
Q Q C T G L O R I O U S
Q G K Z M A I W N U T E
C B Q O T S E Y E S P D
D J X F W O W T D R P Z
```

SHOUT	POWER	RULES
SING	BOWS	FOREVER
GLORIOUS	MANKIND	EYES
AWESOME	TURNED	WATCH
DEEDS	PASSED	REBELLIOUS

Answer on Page 106

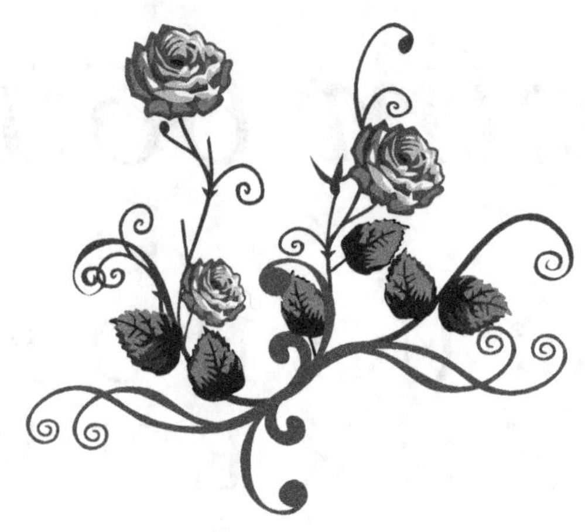

5   You, LORD, are forgiving and good,
      abounding in love to all who call to you.
6   Hear my prayer, LORD;
      listen to my cry for mercy.
7   When I am in distress, I call to you,
      because you answer me.

8   Among the gods there is none like you, LORD;
      no deeds can compare with yours.
9   All the nations you have made
      will come and worship before you, LORD;
      they will bring glory to your name.
10 For you are great and do marvelous deeds;
      you alone are GOD.

Psalm 86:5-10

Psalm 86:5-10

U	M	W	N	A	K	F	C	Z	X	X	T
C	A	L	L	W	D	V	K	F	S	E	O
B	R	D	L	O	V	E	B	X	J	M	G
K	V	I	P	R	A	Y	E	R	H	N	O
U	E	S	I	S	X	I	Q	D	I	L	O
W	L	T	I	H	F	U	W	D	S	N	D
F	O	R	G	I	V	I	N	G	I	G	G
D	U	E	K	P	H	U	A	C	H	B	X
T	S	S	I	C	O	M	P	A	R	E	Q
X	W	S	T	B	V	H	G	A	H	Y	Q
C	R	N	A	L	O	N	E	K	I	A	J
Q	I	F	O	Q	M	H	S	A	V	U	K

FORGIVING	HEAR	WORSHIP
GOOD	PRAYER	BRING
LOVE	CRY	MARVELOUS
ABOUNDING	DISTRESS	DEEDS
CALL	COMPARE	ALONE

Answer on Page 106

1 Whoever dwells in the shelter of the Most High
   will rest in the shadow of the Almighty.
2 I will say of the LORD, "He is my refuge and my
   fortress, my GOD, in whom I trust."

3 Surely he will save you
     from the fowler's snare
     and from the deadly pestilence.
4 He will cover you with his feathers,
     and under his wings you will find refuge;
     his faithfulness will be your shield and rampart.
5 You will not fear the terror of night,
     nor the arrow that flies by day

Psalm 91:1-5

Psalm 91:1-5

```
M I S G W B A Q M A W D
W N U M V D W K X N F R
W F L R F Z M U S Y O S
I E K G W H O E V E R Y
N S C O R E F U G E T T
G U H S A J R F H H R R
S R A M P A R T G E E U
H E R E S T A I T L S S
I L R F E E M L W Z S T
E Y O T F L E O A E P M
L D W E A H F F I P Z N
D R L K S H A D O W J K
```

WHOEVER	REFUGE	FEATHERS
SHELTER	FORTRESS	WINGS
REST	TRUST	SHIELD
SHADOW	SURELY	RAMPART
ALMIGHTY	FOWLER	ARROW

Answer on Page 106

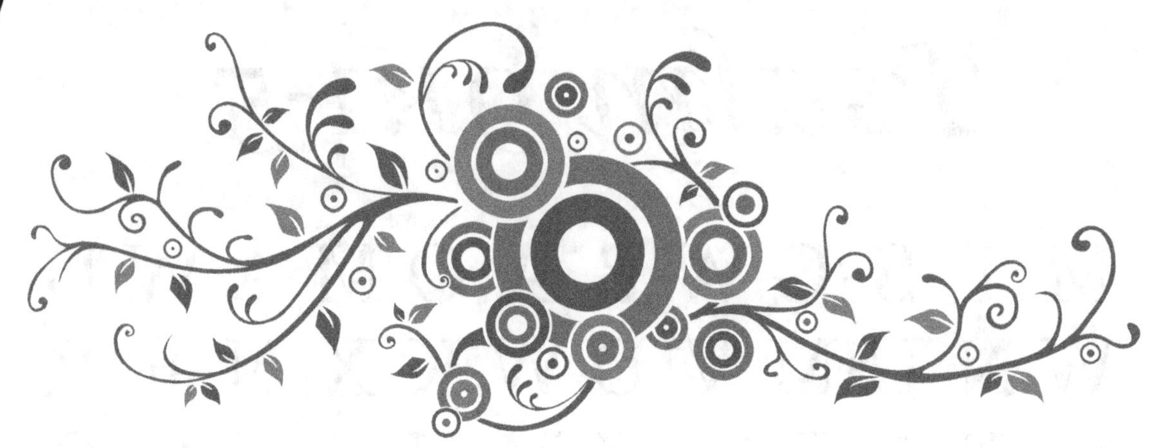

1 Come, let us sing for joy to the LORD;
  let us shout aloud to the Rock of our salvation.
2 Let us come before him with thanksgiving
  and extol him with music and song.

3 For the Lord is the great GOD,
  the great King above all gods.
4 In his hand are the depths of the earth,
  and the mountain peaks belong to him.
5 The sea is his, for he made it,
  and his hands formed the dry land.

6 Come, let us bow down in worship,
  let us kneel before the LORD our Maker

Psalm 95:1-6

Psalm 95:1-6

T	H	A	N	K	S	G	I	V	I	N	G
U	D	R	Y	L	A	N	D	B	X	S	R
R	E	Y	F	S	L	X	Y	Q	K	G	E
A	P	I	K	C	V	I	C	A	I	U	A
M	T	P	I	M	A	K	E	R	N	W	T
J	H	G	H	X	T	P	F	O	G	L	V
X	S	J	R	F	I	B	I	C	I	Z	P
C	W	N	T	H	O	F	N	K	A	B	R
R	L	V	S	A	N	R	L	N	L	Y	N
V	W	R	W	N	B	D	M	E	O	W	I
J	O	Y	R	D	T	G	A	E	U	K	H
W	K	U	G	S	Z	W	E	L	D	M	R

JOY	KING	FORMED
ALOUD	THANKSGIVING	DRY LAND
ROCK	DEPTHS	WORSHIP
SALVATION	PEAKS	KNEEL
GREAT	HANDS	MAKER

24 The LORD has done it this very day;
  let us rejoice today and be glad.

25 LORD, save us!
  LORD, grant us success!

26 Blessed is he who comes in the name of the LORD.
  From the house of the LORD we bless you.
27 The LORD is GOD,
  and he has made his light shine on us.
  With boughs in hand, join in the festal procession
  up to the horns of the altar.

28 You are my GOD, and I will praise you;
  you are my GOD, and I will exalt you.

29 Give thanks to the LORD, for he is good;
  his love endures forever.

Psalm 118:24-29

Psalm 118:24-29

P	R	O	C	E	S	S	I	O	N	B	F
Z	N	U	D	H	U	A	M	Q	C	F	K
Y	P	D	E	J	C	D	T	I	J	O	B
L	S	X	N	U	C	O	O	M	G	R	U
J	O	I	G	Q	E	N	D	U	R	E	S
O	F	H	O	U	S	E	A	S	A	V	E
F	K	I	M	H	S	K	Y	L	N	E	X
E	O	J	G	S	O	F	D	O	T	R	J
L	M	U	E	Y	U	R	P	J	M	A	M
Y	O	L	I	G	H	T	N	H	B	V	R
B	B	V	S	P	D	Y	H	S	T	G	M
D	Q	A	E	Q	P	F	G	A	K	K	O

DONE	BLESSED	ALTAR
TODAY	HOUSE	BOUGHS
SAVE	LIGHT	LOVE
GRANT	PROCESSION	ENDURES
SUCCESS	HORNS	FOREVER

Answer on Page 107

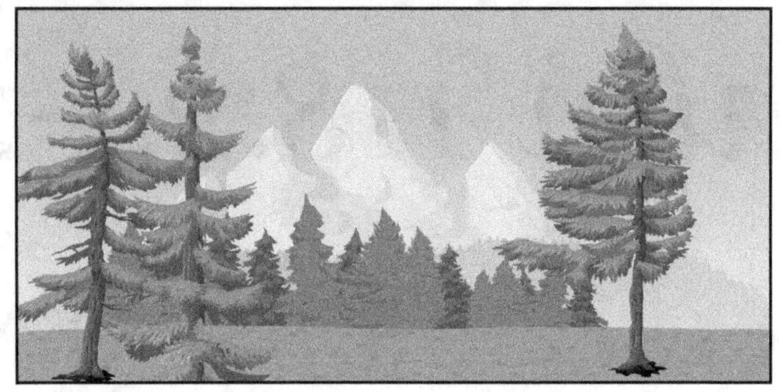

1 I lift up my eyes to the mountains—
  where does my help come from?
2 My help comes from the LORD,
  the Maker of heaven and earth.

3 He will not let your foot slip—
  he who watches over you will not slumber;
4 indeed, he who watches over Israel
  will neither slumber nor sleep.

5 The LORD watches over you—
  the LORD is your shade at your right hand;
6 the sun will not harm you by day,
  nor the moon by night.

7 The LORD will keep you from all harm—
  he will watch over your life;
8 the LORD will watch over your coming and going
  both now and forevermore.

Psalm 121

Psalm 121

S	A	R	E	V	N	E	F	N	L	E	H
Q	A	C	D	V	D	W	N	G	R	T	E
L	H	N	D	Q	P	X	F	O	I	L	L
S	Y	U	M	Y	O	S	M	I	G	S	P
V	B	W	D	P	K	R	T	N	H	U	R
M	Y	P	Q	W	E	R	I	G	T	N	C
J	I	J	N	V	E	M	W	F	H	F	L
A	N	O	E	B	O	S	I	K	A	O	H
A	O	R	M	C	E	L	H	V	N	O	W
M	O	U	N	T	A	I	N	S	D	T	Q
F	L	H	K	E	E	P	J	J	F	M	H
S	H	A	D	E	K	B	R	D	V	E	E

LIFT UP	SLUMBER	KEEP
HELP	SHADE	COMING
MOUNTAINS	RIGHT HAND	GOING
FOOT	SUN	NOW
SLIP	MOON	FOREVERMORE

Answer on Page 107

1 When the LORD restored the fortunes of Zion,
  we were like those who dreamed.
2 Our mouths were filled with laughter,
  our tongues with songs of joy.
  Then it was said among the nations,
  "The LORD has done great things for them."
3 The LORD has done great things for us,
  and we are filled with joy.

4 Restore our fortunes, LORD,
  like streams in the Negev.
5 Those who sow with tears
  will reap with songs of joy.
6 Those who go out weeping,
  carrying seed to sow,
  will return with songs of joy,
  carrying sheaves with them.

Psalm 126

Psalm 126

```
L F I L L E D D U G M G
A O C D V T E Y N X P P
U R C A R R Y I N G E F
G T C I O E P G M Q T E
H U S T R E A M S M X I
T N S E E D M M R O A J
E E E W Z I O N E A W W
R S A G Q R N H A D T P
B F V R E F G D P O F A
E V E L S V Z P U M H N
Q T M A T W A R O T A H
I B O F I R W O T C J A
```

RESTORED	AMONG	TEARS
FORTUNES	FILLED	REAP
ZION	STREAMS	WEEPING
DREAMED	NEGEV	CARRYING
LAUGHTER	SOW	SEED

Answer on Page 107

1 Praise the LORD.

   Sing to the LORD a new song,
     his praise in the assembly of his faithful people.

2 Let Israel rejoice in their Maker;
     let the people of Zion be glad in their King.
3 Let them praise his name with dancing
     and make music to him with timbrel and harp.
4 For the LORD takes delight in his people;
     he crowns the humble with victory.
5 Let his faithful people rejoice in this honor
     and sing for joy on their beds.

Psalm 149:1-5

Psalm 149:1-5

H	Y	R	D	M	E	C	M	L	I	F	U
N	T	D	A	C	W	K	C	P	Y	O	G
B	F	Q	N	F	B	Y	R	R	K	N	Z
E	V	A	C	E	S	A	O	A	O	S	T
D	E	L	I	G	H	T	W	S	Z	Q	M
M	M	O	N	T	C	W	N	S	O	A	J
I	U	R	G	I	H	Y	S	E	F	E	H
H	S	D	V	M	N	F	A	M	J	R	U
O	I	R	W	B	V	G	U	B	Z	O	M
N	C	L	A	R	B	E	G	L	A	D	B
O	A	O	V	E	C	U	Q	Y	G	M	L
R	K	B	L	L	L	C	O	Z	B	E	E

LORD   BE GLAD   DELIGHT
SONG   DANCING   CROWNS
ASSEMBLY   TIMBREL   HUMBLE
FAITHFUL   HARP   VICTORY
ISRAEL   MUSIC   HONOR

Answer on Page 107

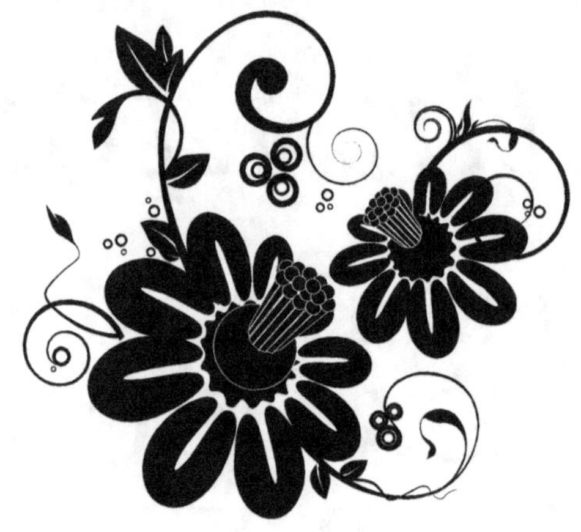

1 Praise the LORD.

   Praise GOD in his sanctuary;
   praise him in his mighty heavens.
2 Praise him for his acts of power;
   praise him for his surpassing greatness.
3 Praise him with the sounding of the trumpet,
   praise him with the harp and lyre,
4 praise him with timbrel and dancing,
   praise him with the strings and pipe,
5 praise him with the clash of cymbals,
   praise him with resounding cymbals.

6 Let everything that has breath praise the LORD.

Praise the LORD.

Psalm 150

Psalm 150

Y	S	M	U	G	H	C	W	U	I	Y	W
S	P	T	B	R	E	A	T	H	G	C	H
G	O	R	B	O	Y	B	R	N	H	Y	A
R	W	U	Y	S	U	P	I	P	E	M	L
E	E	M	N	U	L	S	C	Y	V	B	T
A	R	P	Z	D	S	V	T	L	W	A	N
T	Q	E	X	A	I	H	G	D	A	L	R
N	O	T	P	F	G	N	P	J	P	S	O
E	P	R	A	I	S	E	G	O	D	E	H
S	U	H	M	T	W	P	W	V	R	Q	F
S	A	N	C	T	U	A	R	Y	X	Q	X
T	E	A	S	E	Z	N	L	G	W	J	T

PRAISE GOD   PIPE   BREATH

MIGHTY   SURPASSING   HARP

ACTS   CLASH   GREATNESS

SANCTUARY   LYRE   POWER

TRUMPET   SOUNDING   CYMBALS

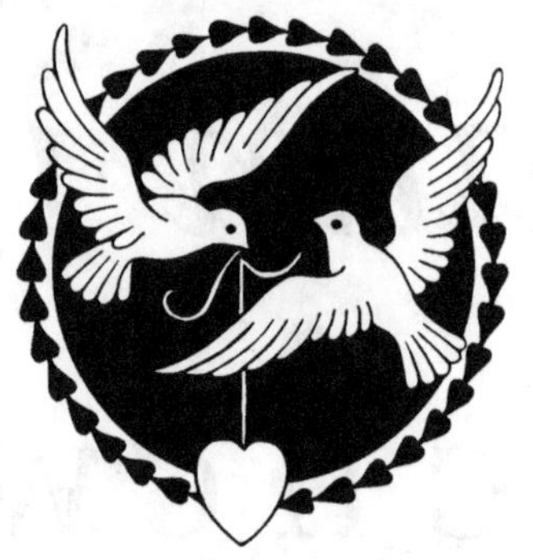

Amazing Grace, how sweet the sound
That saved a wretch like me
I once was lost but now am found
Was blind, but now, I see.

'Twas grace that taught my heart to fear,
And grace my fears relieved;
How precious did that grace appear
The hour I first believed!

The Lord hath promised good to me,
His word my hope secures;
He will my shield and portion be
As long as life endures.

When we've been there ten thousand years,
Bright shining as the sun,
We've no less days to sing God's praise
Than when we first begun.

Amazing Grace

Amazing Grace

```
K A N N P S K S B T T F
B X Z M W E Z X A M P B
C H E H P M M K M V R D
N F N O L P G R A C E N
Y S H I N I N G Z S C D
W R E T C H E F I S I N
B S P C I M K M N H O N
R P H O U N O T G I U B
I E N D U R E S T E S D
G N A G P E E R S L Q C
H B E V W K O S P D J W
T B C S Q P L O I B M M
```

AMAZING   HOPE   PORTION
GRACE   PRECIOUS   ENDURES
SWEET   PROMISED   BRIGHT
SAVED   SECURES   SHINING
WRETCH   SHIELD   BEGUN

Answer on Page 108

Holy, holy, holy! Lord God Almighty!
Early in the morning our song shall rise to Thee;
Holy, holy, holy, merciful and mighty!
God in three Persons, blessed Trinity!

Holy, holy, holy! All the saints adore Thee,
Casting down their golden crowns around the glassy sea,
Cherubim and seraphim falling down before Thee,
Who wert and art, and evermore shalt be.

Holy, holy, holy! Though the darkness hide Thee,
Though the eye of sinful man Thy glory may not see;
Only Thou art holy; there is none beside Thee,
Perfect in power, love, and purity.

Holy, holy, holy! Lord God Almighty!
All Thy works shall praise
Thy name in earth and sky and sea;
Holy, holy, holy, merciful and mighty!
God in three Persons, blessed Trinity!

Holy Holy Holy

Holy Holy Holy

U	C	P	H	Y	G	S	V	B	F	M	U
G	R	K	Q	R	T	R	I	N	I	T	Y
L	O	V	E	N	O	N	O	H	R	F	G
V	W	L	I	T	E	T	P	V	F	F	H
X	N	A	D	H	C	A	F	M	Y	A	U
T	S	Z	M	E	R	C	I	F	U	L	K
G	V	Z	F	E	N	B	N	M	U	L	H
I	X	R	S	P	U	E	J	I	F	I	Y
Y	E	M	O	R	N	I	N	G	U	N	M
P	O	W	E	R	P	Z	U	H	M	G	D
Q	S	H	M	N	Z	N	H	T	U	O	T
A	C	K	T	Q	H	O	L	Y	G	C	A

HOLY
MORNING
MERCIFUL
MIGHTY
TRINITY

SAINTS
GOLDEN
CROWNS
CHERUBIM
SERAPHIM

FALLING
THEE
PERFECT
POWER
LOVE

Answer on Page 108

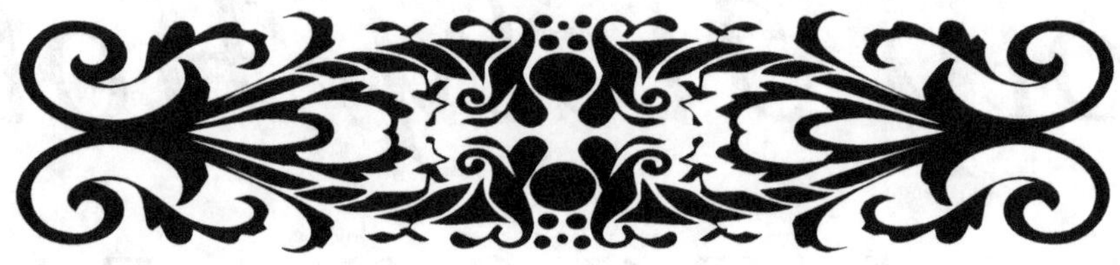

How firm a foundation, ye saints of the Lord,
Is laid for your faith in His excellent word!
What more can He say than to you He hath said,
To you who for refuge to Jesus have fled?

"Fear not, I am with thee, O be not dismayed,
For I am thy God, and will still give thee aid;
I'll strengthen thee, help thee, and cause thee to stand,
Upheld by My righteous, omnipotent hand."

"When through the deep waters I call thee to go,
The rivers of sorrow shall not overflow;
For I will be with thee, thy troubles to bless,
And sanctify to thee thy deepest distress."

"When through fiery trials thy pathway shall lie,
My grace, all sufficient, shall be thy supply;
The flame shall not hurt thee; I only design
Thy dross to consume, and thy gold to refine."

How Firm A Foundation

How Firm A Foundation

```
W O V E R F L O W S A S
K C Q X E A L M W N I U
C A L C F I W N O Y R P
E G P E U T F I R M D P
O L O L G H T P D R E L
Y B F L E A S O K R L Y
M U A E D C W T W A A V
W I X N A P V E C W I F
R V U T R R N N H U D D
K O T L O K N T Y H Q W
F I K J B W A O F B Z C
Z U Y K T P P F T Y G D
```

FIRM	WORD	OVERFLOW
FOUNDATION	REFUGE	CALL
LAID	FEAR NOT	PATHWAY
FAITH	AID	SUPPLY
EXCELLENT	OMNIPOTENT	GOLD

Answer on Page 108

Come, Thou Fount of every blessing,
Tune my heart to sing Thy grace;
Streams of mercy, never ceasing,
Call for songs of loudest praise.
Jesus sought me when a stranger,
Wand'ring from the face of God;
He, to save my soul from danger,
Interposed His precious blood.

O to grace how great a debtor
Daily I'm constrained to be!
Let that grace, Lord, like a fetter,
Bind my wand'ring heart to Thee.
Teach me, Lord, some rapturous measure,
Meet for me Thy grace to prove,
While I sing the countless treasure
Of my God's unchanging love.

Come Thou Fount of Every Blessing

Come Thou Fount of Every Blessing

```
E Q I F G L F G E N P B
V Q E P T G O R X U R G
S C Q R Z U U A V J E Z
M M R O R S N C L B C L
E G E V A T T E O L I Z
R E S E P R F C U E O G
C Z R O T A G X D S U H
Y T C O U N T L E S S L
D U B G R G P T S I L Y
Q F E L O E H J T N W M
E H L X U R T T U G Y Z
Z A F A S B L O O D J C
```

FOUNT	LOUDEST	TREASURE
BLESSING	SOUGHT	RAPTUROUS
TUNE	STRANGER	PROVE
GRACE	PRECIOUS	COUNTLESS
MERCY	BLOOD	MEET

Answer on Page 109

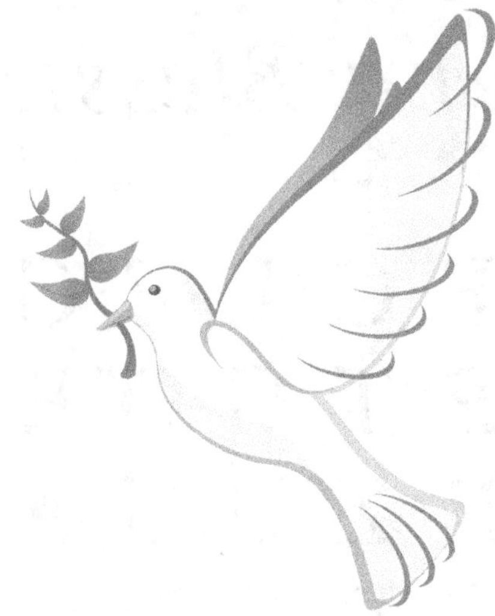

When peace like a river attendeth my way,
When sorrows like sea billows roll;
Whatever my lot Thou hast taught me to say,
"It is well, it is well with my soul!"
It is well with my soul!
It is well, it is well with my soul!

Though Satan should buffet, though
trials should come,
Let this blessed assurance control,
That Christ hath regarded my helpless estate,
And hath shed His own blood for my soul.

It Is Well

It Is Well

```
E B W R C J A A M O S Z
T I B O P H B C B T O L
C L C O N T R O L D U D
T L E Z Y K H I E O E T
R O A S P P E D S H X K
I W T Q T E R R S T R H
A S S U R A N C E C U H
L P W E G C T F D I C Q
S B V E D E F E G Q G I
L I R V L U M K V W U O
R O L L B L Z J S W W O
M N F W R Z F I J H Z L
```

PEACE	BUFFET	CHRIST
IS WELL	TRIALS	REGARDED
BILLOWS	BLESSED	ESTATE
ROLL	ASSURANCE	SHED
SOUL	CONTROL	RIVER

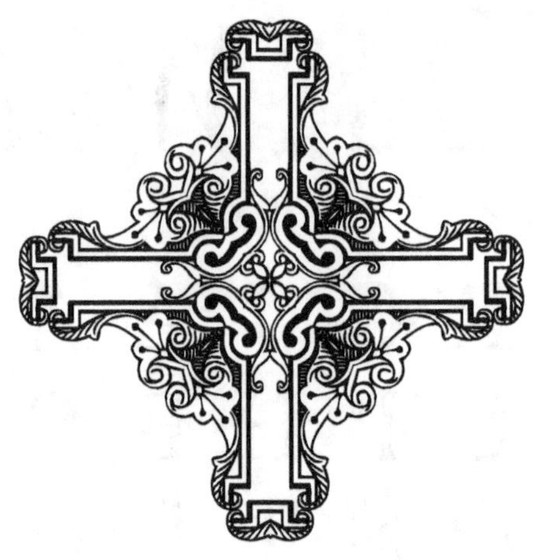

Praise to the Lord, the Almighty,
the King of creation!
O my soul, praise Him, for He is thy
health and salvation!
All ye who hear,
Now to His temple draw near;
Sing now in glad adoration!

Praise to the Lord, who o'er all
things so wondrously reigneth,
Who, as on wings of an eagle,
uplifteth, sustaineth.
Hast thou not seen
How thy desires all have been
Granted in what He ordaineth?

Praise to the Lord
the Almighty

Praise to the Lord the Almighty

```
M F N Q Y C F T W E I Q
Z E P T E W S G I H L E
P R J O R D A I N E T H
Q E C E A G L E G A K R
E S D S Z T V J S L A V
O T B Z J A A D B T A E
V U P L I F T E T H L D
A D O R A T I O N P J X
C R E A T I O N M D V D
S U S T A I N E T H S O
A L M I G H T Y K I N G
R E I G N E T H E A R M
```

ALMIGHTY	SALVATION	UPLIFTETH
KING	GLAD	ORDAINETH
CREATION	ADORATION	EAGLE
HEALTH	REIGNETH	WINGS
TEMPLE	HEAR	SUSTAINETH

Answer on Page 109

Be Thou my vision, O Lord of my heart;
Naught be all else to me, save that Thou art;
Thou my best thought, by day or by night;
Waking or sleeping, Thy presence my light.

Be Thou my wisdom, and Thou my true Word;
I ever with Thee and Thou with me, Lord;
Thou my great Father and I, Thy true son;
Thou in me dwelling, and I with Thee one.

Riches I heed not, nor man's empty praise;
Thou mine inheritance, now and always;
Thou and Thou only, first in my heart;
O King of glory, my treasure Thou art.

O King of glory, my victory won;
Rule and reign in me 'til Thy will be done;
Heart of my own heart, whatever befall;
Still be my vision, O Ruler of all.

Be Thou My Vision

Be Thou My Vision

```
I N H E R I T A N C E F
F S L I G H T H I C J S
A A O D G A Z G N B X O
B V E U W N N E U M F F
D E O G V I S I O N Q U
H H F J K E S O B G Y D
T H E A R T R D G R E G
L W W P L E L N O S D W
B X Y R L L I L Y M X T
X M G U S K G G A O X E
W P R A I E D O N J H W
W F K O L G R I E J I B
```

VISION	PRESENCE	KING
HEART	LIGHT	GLORY
THOUGHT	WISDOM	REIGN
SAVE	INHERITANCE	BEFALL
WAKING	HEED	RULER

Answer on Page 109

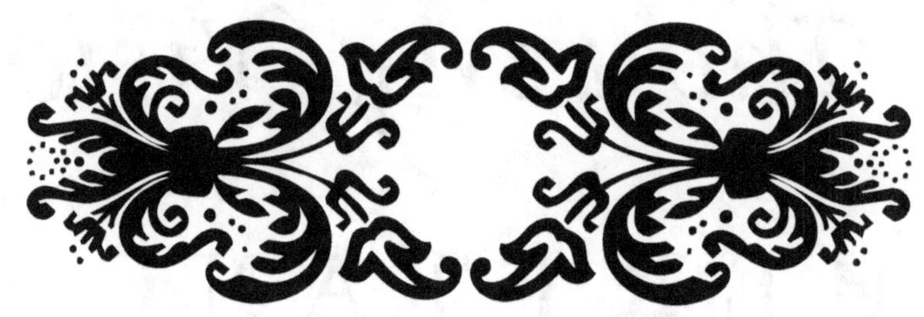

All creatures of our God and King
Lift up your voice and with us sing
O praise Him! Alleluia!
Thou, burning sun with golden beam
Thou, silver moon with softer gleam
O praise Him! O praise Him!
Alleluia! Alleluia! Alleluia!

Let all things their Creator bless
And worship Him in humbleness
O praise Him! Alleluia!
Praise, praise the Father, praise the Son
And praise the Spirit, Three-in-One
O praise Him! O praise Him!
Alleluia! Alleluia! Alleluia!

*All Creatures of Our
God and King*

All Creatures of Our God and King

```
F H Q N X W K A T P K Y
A B Q V D D O H A W W F
T L I F T Z K R D I X S
I E L T O X B Z S V V N
O S K E U A U E O H O O
P S I B L M R F Y S I L
G I N S H U N E M A C P
C L G F T K I G N O E K
B V L A A V N A D Q O S
E E E H M I G O L D E N
P R A I S E T I I J W X
C M M M L E L F P R X Z
```

LIFT	ALLELUIA	GLEAM
CREATURES	BEAM	MOON
KING	GOLDEN	BLESS
HIM	BURNING	WORSHIP
PRAISE	SILVER	VOICE

Answer on Page 110

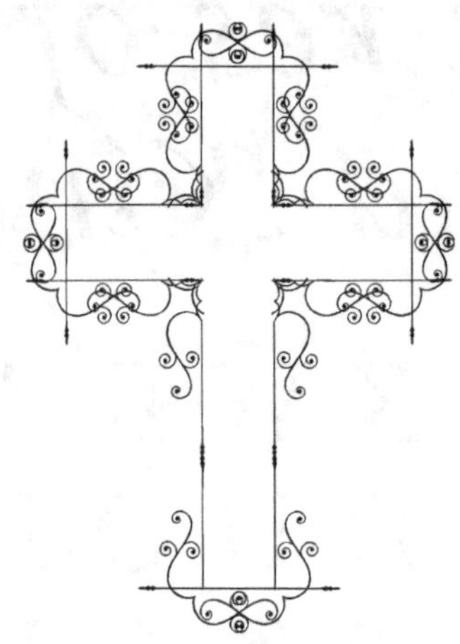

All hail the power of Jesus' name!
Let angels prostrate fall,
Let angels prostrate fall;
Bring forth the royal diadem,
And crown Him, crown Him,
crown Him, crown Him;
And crown Him Lord of all!

Ye chosen seed of Israel's race,
Ye ransomed from the fall,
Ye ransomed from the fall,
Hail Him who saves you by His grace

*All Hail the Power
of Jesus' Name*

All Hail the Power of Jesus' Name

I	T	B	L	Q	L	D	X	J	S	U	B
N	N	P	O	R	A	K	B	X	Y	M	U
Q	N	R	A	N	S	O	M	E	D	N	I
F	T	O	N	Y	F	P	T	O	I	O	B
B	G	Y	G	N	E	A	O	H	A	I	L
D	Y	A	E	Z	R	J	L	W	D	S	Z
C	B	L	L	T	O	E	M	L	E	B	D
Q	H	C	S	F	A	S	S	V	M	R	M
H	Q	O	K	R	T	U	A	M	O	I	D
I	R	B	S	L	O	S	U	L	L	N	E
P	K	I	M	E	F	Q	B	L	W	G	A
K	C	R	O	W	N	V	B	Z	K	U	D

HAIL	DIADEM	POWER
JESUS	ROYAL	RANSOMED
PROSTRATE	CHOSEN	BRING
FALL	ISRAEL	LORD
ANGELS	CROWN	SAVES

Answer on Page 110

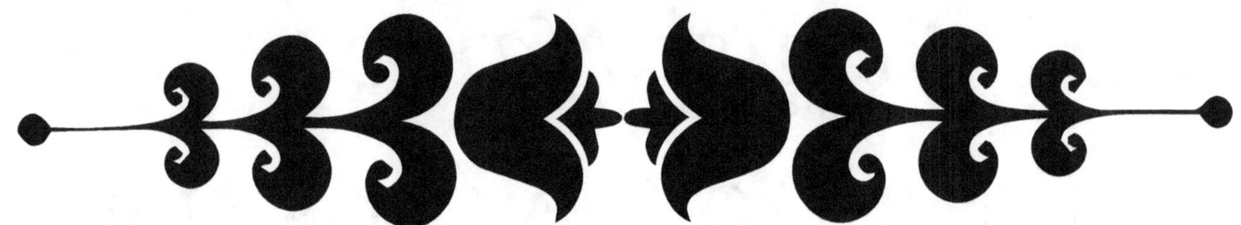

To God be the glory, great things He hath done,
So loved He the world that He gave us His Son,
Who yielded His life our redemption to win,
And opened the life-gate that all may go in.

Praise the Lord, praise the Lord,
Let the earth hear His voice;
Praise the Lord, praise the Lord,
Let the people rejoice;

Oh, come to the Father, through Jesus the Son,
And give Him the glory;
great things He hath done.

To God Be the Glory

To God Be the Glory

U	H	P	O	D	G	I	R	F	X	B	M
F	F	L	O	S	Z	A	J	M	H	F	B
A	P	G	O	D	G	I	T	N	J	I	Z
R	R	Y	G	V	T	A	B	E	N	J	G
P	E	O	P	L	E	A	R	T	H	Y	D
S	J	P	N	R	O	D	X	G	A	C	L
Q	O	E	G	V	N	R	A	H	R	W	H
W	I	N	A	K	X	W	Y	E	S	H	L
B	C	E	V	R	M	V	H	P	I	W	D
R	E	D	E	M	P	T	I	O	N	L	Y
R	C	D	W	P	A	A	D	R	E	Q	I
Z	D	K	I	F	C	R	U	B	N	N	I

GOD	REDEMPTION	EARTH
GLORY	SON	PEOPLE
LOVED	OPENED	GREAT
GAVE	GATE	FATHER
ONLY	WIN	REJOICE

Answer on Page 110

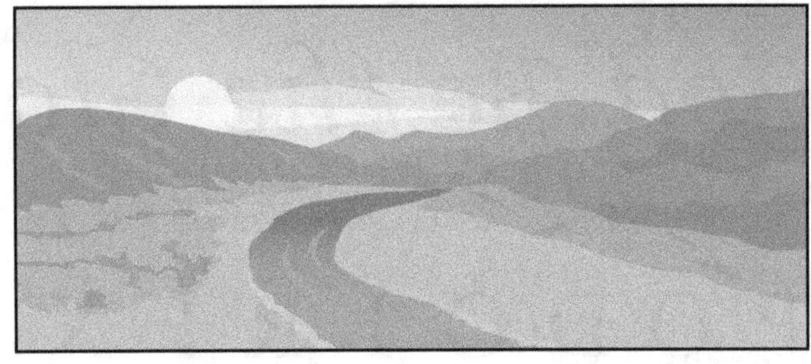

In the sweet by and by
We shall meet on that beautiful shore
In the sweet by and by
Oh, we shall meet on that beautiful shore

There's a land that is fairer than day
And by faith we can see it a-far
For the Father waits over the way
To prepare us a dwelling place there

In the sweet by and by
We shall meet on that beautiful shore
In the sweet by and by
We shall meet on that beautiful shore

We shall sing on that beautiful shore
The melodious songs of the blessed
And their spirits shall sorrow no more
Not a sigh for the blessings of rest

In the Sweet By-and-By

In the Sweet By-and-By

```
O H Z B L E S S I N G S
G V I P G D W U S X U M
W S B Q E O B A P O W S
K S Z B E A U T I F U L
J L M N Y R W D R T R L
Y F P E E A O A I H S S
S H O R E L N Y T E Y N
P G I C E T Y D S W L W
L A V M X P V P B A A N
F A T H E R A V R Y O S
J A N K L J Y R Y I P J
G W E D E S W E E T J T
```

SWEET	LAND	THE WAY
BY AND BY	DAY	MELODIOUS
MEET	FAIRER	SPIRITS
SHORE	FATHER	BLESSINGS
BEAUTIFUL	WAITS	PREPARE

Answer on Page 110

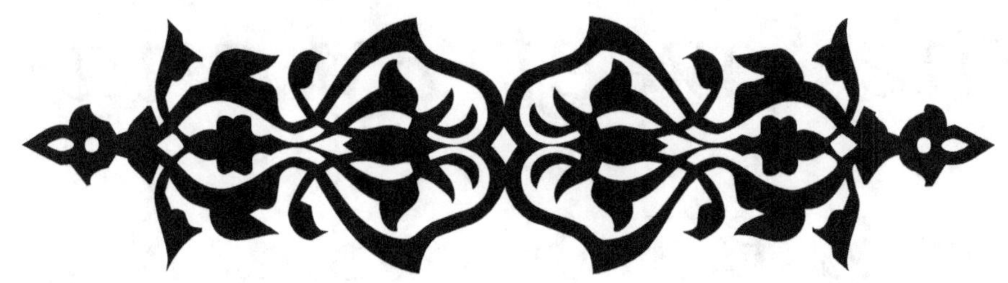

What a Friend we have in Jesus,
All our sins and griefs to bear!
What a privilege to carry
Everything to God in prayer!
O what peace we often forfeit,
O what needless pain we bear,
All because we do not carry
Everything to God in prayer!

Have we trials and temptations?
Is there trouble anywhere?
We should never be discouraged,
Take it to the Lord in prayer.
Can we find a friend so faithful
Who will all our sorrows share?
Jesus knows our every weakness,
Take it to the Lord in prayer.

*What A Friend We
Have in Jesus*

What A Friend We Have in Jesus

M	L	K	F	H	C	P	Z	N	N	R	N
G	T	R	O	U	B	L	E	N	H	S	C
C	R	X	R	V	D	G	J	A	H	W	G
J	T	I	F	N	E	G	Y	Q	C	B	E
U	S	R	E	L	P	R	H	A	V	E	G
P	O	I	I	F	R	S	G	G	N	A	U
T	R	I	T	A	S	I	X	B	Y	R	Z
F	R	A	C	Q	L	N	N	S	F	A	A
P	O	X	Y	J	E	S	U	S	F	C	U
A	W	C	N	E	B	Y	W	M	E	O	R
I	S	Z	D	Z	R	H	L	O	D	H	L
N	E	F	M	W	U	F	B	U	H	Y	B

FRIEND	BEAR	TRIALS
HAVE	CARRY	FORFEIT
JESUS	PRIILEGE	PEACE
SINS	PRAYER	TROUBLE
GRIEFS	PAIN	SORROWS

Answer on Page 111

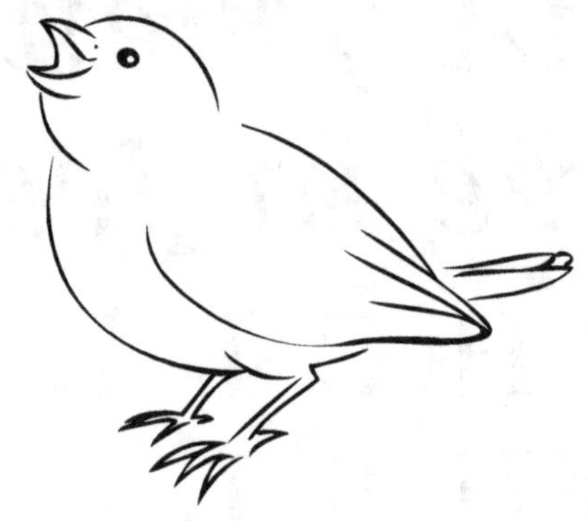

Why should I feel discouraged,
why should the shadows come,
Why should my heart be lonely,
and long for heaven and home,

When Jesus is my portion?
My constant friend is He:
His eye is on the sparrow,
and I know He watches me;
His eye is on the sparrow,
and I know He watches me.

I sing because I'm happy,
I sing because I'm free,
For His eye is on the sparrow,
And I know He watches me.

His Eye Is on the Sparrow

His Eye Is on the Sparrow

V	W	H	O	Y	H	E	B	M	Q	H	A
U	S	H	U	H	E	A	R	T	C	R	L
U	I	C	E	M	E	Y	E	V	Q	V	Y
V	M	S	O	K	H	A	P	P	Y	D	Y
S	E	H	P	N	F	W	V	N	N	U	V
H	V	A	W	A	S	F	R	E	E	H	T
A	F	J	P	O	R	T	I	O	N	P	X
D	I	S	C	O	U	R	A	G	E	D	S
O	J	A	J	U	F	L	O	N	E	L	Y
W	A	T	C	H	E	S	W	W	T	T	Z
S	T	J	W	R	E	G	I	C	H	P	J
D	E	F	A	Z	L	G	X	I	B	E	S

SPARROW   PORTION   CONSTANT

FEEL   HOME   EYE

DISCOURAGED   HEAVEN   WATCHES

HEART   SHADOWS   FREE

LONELY   FRIEND   HAPPY

Answer on Page 111

Mine eyes have seen the glory of the coming of the Lord;
He is trampling out the vintage where
the grapes of wrath are stored;
He hath loosed the fateful lightning of
His terrible swift sword;
His truth is marching on.

Glory! Glory! Hallelujah!
Glory! Glory! Hallelujah!
Glory! Glory! Hallelujah!
His truth is marching on.

He has sounded forth the trumpet
that shall never call retreat;
He is sifting out the hearts of men before His judgment seat;
Oh, be swift, my soul, to answer Him; be jubilant, my feet!
Our God is marching on.

Battle Hymn of the Republic

Battle Hymn of the Republic

```
G M O Q N W G F L M L R
T A K T I L G A L Z E W
K R J R E X D R M H Y U
F C A U V I N T A G E D
Q H M M B E R J R P S K
N I S P P I U Z C U E Z
F N N E C L L V H N T S
U G I T E O I A I A F H
B M N L N N M N N O A Y
O M L K U J N I G T P M
B A T T L E O T N F D N
H L I G H T N I N G X Z
```

EYES	TRAMPLING	MARCHING
SEEN	GRAPES	HALLELUJAH
COMING	VINTAGE	TRUMPET
BATTLE	LIGHTNING	JUBILANT
HYMN	TRUTH	MARCHING

Answer on Page 111

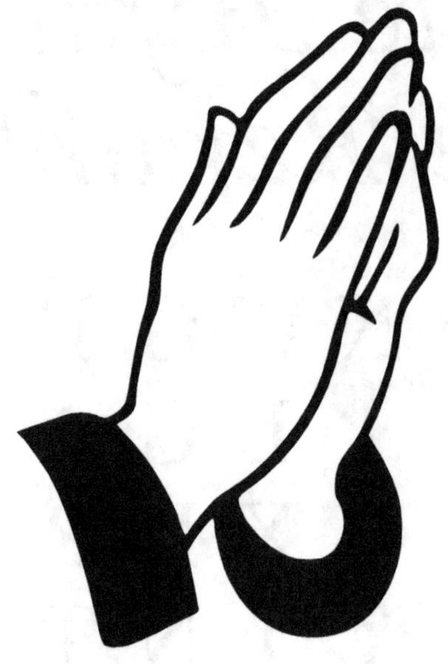

As I went down in the valley to pray,
Studying about that good old way;
You shall wear the starry crown,
Good Lord, show me the way.

By-and-by we'll all go down,
all go down, all go down,
By-and-by we'll all go down,
Down in the valley to pray.

Come, Let Us All Go Down

Come, Let Us All Go Down

U	W	P	C	C	J	A	W	I	X	D	K
P	V	R	Y	M	K	O	L	O	R	D	M
S	T	A	R	R	Y	Q	Q	L	K	S	M
J	Z	Y	L	X	H	W	S	M	G	H	U
D	I	G	Z	L	E	T	U	S	O	O	E
K	B	P	G	K	E	M	C	R	O	W	N
L	W	D	D	M	J	Y	I	N	D	U	X
X	D	Q	O	H	S	B	I	P	I	S	E
H	X	C	A	W	E	A	R	M	F	I	L
L	S	N	A	A	N	Z	O	L	V	R	U
G	E	U	F	K	K	M	C	L	W	T	V
A	C	S	C	O	X	K	Z	I	C	O	I

COME	PRAY	GOOD
ALL GO	VALLEY	LORD
DOWN	LET US	SHOW US
STARRY	WEAR	CROWN

Shall we gather at the river,
Where bright angel feet have trod,
With its crystal tide forever
Flowing by the throne of God?

Yes, we'll gather at the river,
The beautiful, the beautiful river;
Gather with the saints at the river
That flows by the throne of God.

On the margin of the river,
Washing up its silver spray,
We will talk and worship ever,
All the happy golden day.

Shall We Gather at the River

Shall We Gather at the River

G	H	H	P	D	U	A	Z	H	A	R	Y	
W	Y	N	W	O	M	H	W	S	G	A	Y	
L	P	K	F	G	V	B	O	A	R	H	Y	
L	A	C	O	L	A	F	R	P	R	L	S	
H	M	G	R	H	O	T	S	I	U	N	A	
I	J	M	E	Y	A	W	H	F	G	T	I	
P	L	F	V	N	S	P	I	E	M	H	N	
R	I	V	E	R	U	T	P	N	R	R	T	
K	F	A	R	I	U	R	A	Y	G	O	S	
U	O	E	S	A	N	G	E	L	G	N	F	
C	B	G	E	J	Z	G	O	L	D	E	N	
T	L	B	G	T	K	S	S	S	F	B	D	

GATHER	CRYSTAL	BEAUTIFUL
RIVER	THRONE	WORSHIP
BRIGHT	FLOWING	SPRAY
ANGEL	FOREVER	HAPPY
FEET	SAINTS	GOLDEN

Answer on Page 112

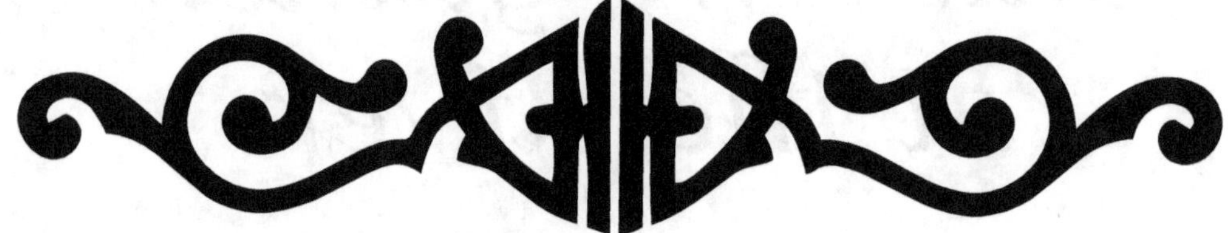

Abide with me; fast falls the eventide;
The darkness deepens; Lord with me abide.
When other helpers fail and comforts flee,
Help of the helpless, O abide with me.

Swift to its close ebbs out life's little day;
Earth's joys grow dim; its glories pass away;
Change and decay in all around I see;
O Thou who changest not, abide with me.

Not a brief glance I beg, a passing word,
But as Thou dwell'st with Thy disciples, Lord,
Familiar, condescending, patient, free.
Come not to sojourn, but abide with me.

Come not in terror, as the King of kings,
But kind and good, with healing in Thy wings;
Tears for all woes, a heart for every plea.
Come, Friend of sinners, thus abide with me.

Abide With Me

Abide With Me

Y	A	N	N	W	J	U	I	O	X	Q	I
E	B	B	S	O	C	C	A	A	A	C	C
O	K	C	I	G	E	M	S	B	F	T	E
D	W	O	R	D	V	S	A	B	H	A	O
U	X	M	X	P	E	T	F	W	S	O	M
V	W	F	C	N	N	X	G	I	O	W	G
Z	C	O	K	E	T	N	A	T	J	I	L
B	H	R	I	E	I	Q	T	H	O	N	A
M	A	T	E	L	D	E	U	M	U	G	N
D	A	S	A	H	E	L	P	E	R	S	C
P	R	E	Y	L	A	C	H	A	N	G	E
U	H	A	F	E	E	B	S	A	A	S	R

ABIDE	FLEE	WORD
WITH ME	HELPERS	PATIENT
EVENTIDE	EBBS	HEALING
DARKNESS	CHANGE	WINGS
COMFORTS	GLANCE	SOJOURN

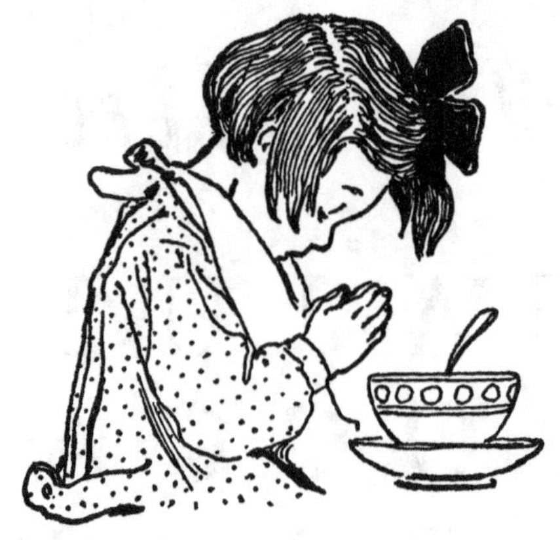

Now thank we all our God,
with heart and hands and voices,
Who wondrous things has done,
in Whom this world rejoices;
Who from our mothers' arms
has blessed us on our way
With countless gifts of love,
and still is ours today.

O may this bounteous God
through all our life be near us,
With ever joyful hearts
and blessed peace to cheer us;
And keep us in His grace,
and guide us when perplexed;
And free us from all ills,
in this world and the next!

Now Thank We All Our God

Now Thank We All Our God

A	W	O	N	D	R	O	U	S	B	L	E
E	Z	X	B	Z	E	U	U	Y	I	D	M
T	T	W	V	L	J	O	Y	F	U	L	L
J	H	W	K	E	E	P	J	J	W	X	T
H	E	A	R	T	E	S	S	H	O	X	L
C	O	U	N	T	L	E	S	S	R	G	W
E	V	U	G	K	C	T	X	E	L	R	L
D	O	Q	I	I	F	C	H	U	D	F	C
B	I	E	O	I	I	T	A	O	Y	F	L
L	C	J	G	Q	O	J	N	V	A	G	O
G	E	N	N	M	T	T	D	L	Z	C	I
R	S	R	N	A	R	M	S	N	H	X	R

THANK	WONDROUS	COUNTLESS
HEART	REJOICES	BLESSED
HANDS	MOTHER	JOYFUL
VOICES	ARMS	BOUNTEOUS
WORLD	GIFTS	KEEP

Answer on Page 112

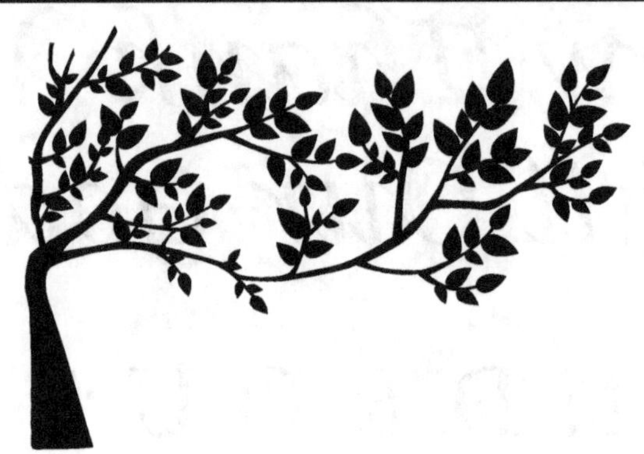

Crown Him with many crowns,
The Lamb upon His throne;
Hark! how the heavenly anthem drowns
All music but its own!
Awake, my soul, and sing
Of Him who died for thee,
And hail Him as thy matchless King
Through all eternity.

Crown Him the Virgin's Son,
The God Incarnate born,
Whose arm those crimson trophies won
Which now His brow adorn:
Fruit of the mystic Tree,
As of that Tree the Stem;
The Root whence flows Thy mercy free,
The Babe of Bethlehem.

Crown Him with Many Crowns

Crown Him with Many Crowns

```
P A C R O W N N D K Y G
L H R S Y N M M M M U L
P Q I B C E F E U Y J V
O I M A T C H L E S S A
R A S S N E E T T T I J
L N O D L B A B E I B C
I T N H M N V H R C Q Z
K H T D R A E C N W B L
H E K A D K N G I X A T
B M C M A Q L Y T Y S B
T N G W J T Y A Y Y C D
I C A M N S L X W Q T Z
```

CROWN	ANTHEM	INCARNATE
MANY	AWAKE	MYSTIC
LAMB	MATCHLESS	STEM
MUSIC	ETERNITY	BETHLEHEM
HEAVENLY	CRIMSON	BABE

Answer on Page 112

If you will only let God guide you,
And hope in Him through all your ways,
Whatever comes, He'll stand beside you,
To bear you through the evil days.
Who trusts in God's unchanging love
Builds on the Rock that cannot move.

2.
Only be still, and wait His leisure
In cheerful hope, with heart content
To take whatever the Father's pleasure
And all discerning love have sent;
Nor doubt our inmost wants are known,
To Him who chose us for His own.

3.
Sing, pray, and swerve not from His ways,
But do your part in conscience true;
Trust His rich promises of grace,
So shall they be fulfilled in you;
God hears the call of those in need,
The souls that trust in Him indeed.

If You Will Only Let God Guide You

If You Will Only Let God Guide You

```
C O N T E N T K G C B U
R O C K R F W S M P X N
F K N X T U U M H O D C
S V J S A L S X S O E H
Z W C I C F C T G B Z A
F T E A S I H T S E R N
D C A R L L E I F S W G
A R L Z V L E N W I X I
X S H O P E R T C D L N
Z S T A N D F H G E J G
H P L E A S U R E D B N
D M O K H G L P R A Y D
```

LET GOD	ROCK	PRAY
STAND	HOPE	CONSCIENCE
BESIDE	CHEERFUL	FULFILLED
TRUSTS	CONTENT	CALL
UNCHANGING	PLEASURE	SWERVE

Answer on Page 113

Blessed assurance, Jesus is mine;
Oh, what a foretaste of glory divine!
Heir of salvation, purchase of God,
Born of His Spirit, washed in His blood.

This is my story, this is my song,
Praising my Savior all the day long.
This is my story, this is my song,
Praising my Savior all the day long.

Perfect submission, perfect delight,
Visions of rapture now burst on my sight;
Angels descending, bring from above
Echoes of mercy, whispers of love.

Blessed Assurance

Blessed Assurance

```
I U D A P M V W T M E M
C A S S U R A N C E A I I
D K A U S I A M B O R N N
X E X B E T D I V I N E E
N I L M O E O P S Q W C
N W H I S P E R S I Z E
W A A S G R I A Y P N S
M L E S O H R P F J O G
Y L Y I H U T T C Y H C
B D V O G E T U B G X O
O A N N F E D R L J T K
S Y O E C H O E S P T D
```

MINE	BORN	SUBMISSION
DIVINE	STORY	DELIGHT
ASSURANCE	PRAISING	RAPTURE
BLESSED	SAVIOR	ECHOES
WASHED	ALL DAY	WHISPERS

Answer on Page 113

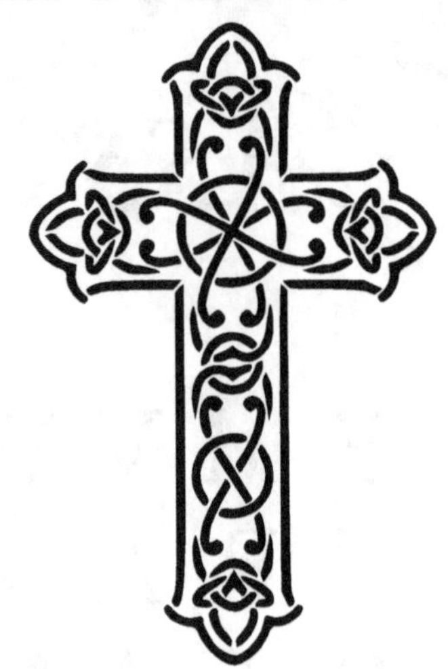

When we survey the wondrous cross
On which the Lord of glory died,
Our richest gain we count but loss,
And pour contempt on all our pride.

Our God forbid that we should boast,
Save in the death of Christ, our Lord;
All the vain things that charm us most,
We'd sacrifice them to His blood.

There from His head, His hands, His feet,
Sorrow and love flowed mingled down;
Did e'er such love and sorrow meet,
Or thorns compose so rich a crown?

When We Survey The Wondrous Cross

When We Survey The Wondrous Cross

A	F	I	P	S	A	B	L	O	O	D	T
Q	O	S	S	R	M	O	O	D	X	J	O
R	J	I	C	D	I	E	D	A	Q	V	T
K	G	G	A	I	N	D	H	D	S	E	D
T	C	Y	N	S	G	L	E	U	A	T	Y
S	H	W	S	S	L	Y	O	U	C	R	J
K	A	O	O	M	E	R	B	Z	R	P	Y
K	R	D	R	V	D	R	W	L	I	T	M
C	M	P	R	N	I	O	Y	P	F	V	C
V	Y	U	O	C	S	K	L	A	I	F	H
U	S	W	W	U	Z	Z	D	K	C	L	G
L	C	E	V	F	R	I	C	H	E	S	T

SURVEY	GAIN	SACRIFICE
WONDROUS	POUR	BLOOD
CROSS	PRIDE	SORROW
DIED	BOAST	THORNS
RICHEST	CHARM	MINGLED

Answer on Page 113

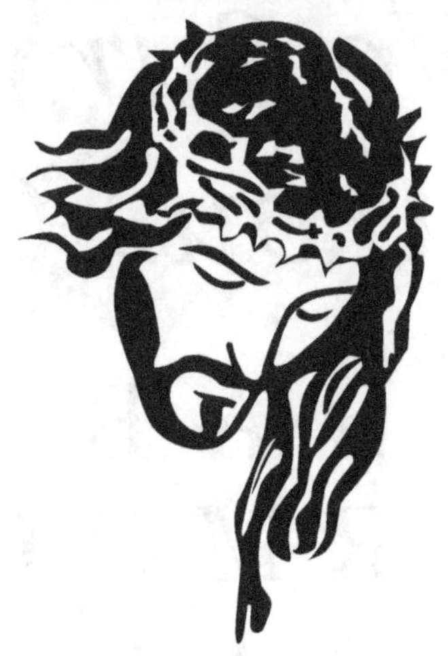

I hear the Savior say,
"Thy strength indeed is small;
Child of weakness, watch and pray,
Find in Me thine all in all."

Jesus paid it all,
All to Him I owe;
Sin had left a crimson stain,
He washed it white as snow.

For nothing good have I
Whereby Thy grace to claim;
I'll wash my garments white
In the blood of Calvary's Lamb.

Jesus Paid It All

Jesus Paid It All

```
G Y Q S W A T C H E E D
C A L V A R Y E Q M G R
W H R Q S V E P W D A V
N E I M H X I P Y L L N
E G A L E Z S O F H M D
X G S K D N W J R A X E
S T R E N G T H B D W O
D U F A H E J S I O D M
L B Z P C H S A N T I S
A W E P R E P S C M E P
V R W J W A T C I W Z J
K E E R O R Y P V A B Y
```

HEAR	WATCH	WHITE
PAID	PRAY	SNOW
SAVIOR	WEAKNESS	GRACE
STRENGTH	OWE	GARMENTS
CHILD	WASHED	CALVARY

Answer on Page 113

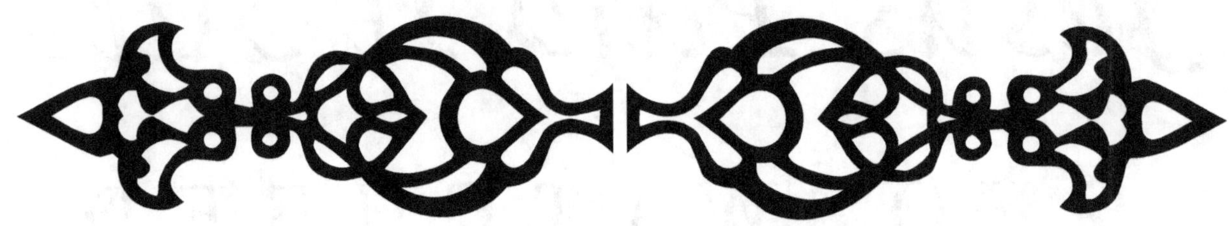

A mighty fortress is our God, a bulwark never failing;
Our helper He, amid the flood of
mortal ills prevailing:
For still our ancient foe doth seek to work us woe;
His craft and power are great,
and, armed with cruel hate,
On earth is not his equal.

And though this world, with devils filled,
should threaten to undo us,
We will not fear, for God hath willed
His truth to triumph through us;
The Prince of Darkness grim,
we tremble not for him;
His rage we can endure, for lo, his doom is sure,
One little word shall fell him.

*A Mighty Fortress
Is Our God*

A Mighty Fortress
Is Our God

I	E	G	E	X	T	F	B	R	G	X	T
M	G	B	N	B	A	R	N	N	G	P	K
E	B	F	D	S	U	E	I	V	G	G	E
M	T	O	U	V	T	L	A	U	J	I	M
C	W	R	R	A	I	L	W	S	M	G	I
R	P	T	E	A	Z	D	H	A	O	P	G
A	X	R	V	M	C	W	E	N	R	U	H
F	H	E	W	X	B	C	L	C	T	K	T
T	R	S	K	O	N	L	P	I	A	C	Y
P	Z	S	M	I	R	I	E	E	L	Q	X
O	R	A	R	M	E	D	R	N	P	K	Z
X	O	P	O	U	Q	Z	D	T	O	K	V

FORTRESS	PREVAILING	TRIUMPH
MIGHTY	ANCIENT	PRINCE
BULWARK	CRAFT	TREMBLE
HELPER	ARMED	ENDURE
MORTAL	THREATEN	WORD

Answer on Page 114

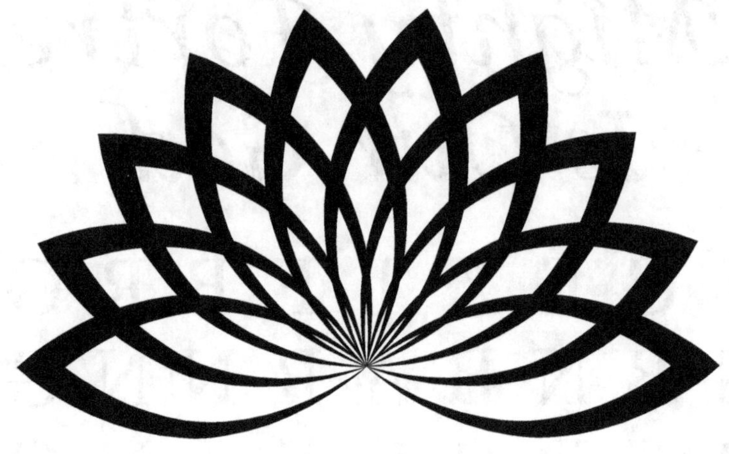

Alas! and did my Savior bleed
And did my Sovereign die?
Would He devote that sacred head
For sinners such as I?

At the cross, at the cross
where I first saw the light,
And the burden of my heart rolled away,
It was there by faith I received my sight,
And now I am happy all the day!

Well might the sun in darkness hide
And shut his glories in,
When Christ, the mighty Maker died,
For man the creature's sin.

At the Cross

At the Cross

```
D P H I S H P M A K E R
M E E E I G X Z T R F Z
C C V J G M M H U O C Q
H E V O H Y G T Z K C J
R C W B T I A P S B Y G
I R O L L E D E I I H N
S O V E R E I G N Z V R
T S D C R R E B R F H S
H S S C O D E D V H I L
N F A L A S L M Q N W O
E S G E Z N L J W A I T
U O H W N T F F C Y L Z
```

CROSS	HEAD	GLORIES
BLEED	SOVEREIGN	CHRIST
ALAS	LIGHT	MAKER
DEVOTE	ROLLED	CREATURE
SACRED	SIGHT	SIN

Answer on Page 114

Answers: Puzzles pages 3-9

Psalm 1

Psalm 4

Psalm 8:5-9

Psalm 13

Answers: Puzzles pages 11-17

M X Z M F K Y J F B U R
D B Y V P S E C U R E I
H R O M E L H Z I C Y S
W F E U I T E A N Q L B
T P A E N I E A K E Q L
X O E I S D T R S E K W
S R N Q T I A N N A N H
S T B G R H U R O A N V
X I H E U O F C Y Z L T
V O H C C E J U F T V G
E N P A T H W P L E I M
I P R E S E N C E Y E S

Psalm 16:5-8

U O V E R W H E L M E D
E N T A N G L E D D S E
S N A R E S A Z S Y T L
S A L V A T I O N W R I
X Z S H I E L D Y R O V
D E S T R U C T I O N E
F O R T R E S S P C G R
P O J I W E F D B K H E
D G B B N J N U T E O R
B Y S R G F H G G C L L
K C O N F R O N T E D B
F H I A E W O R T H Y H

Psalm 18:1-5

H V S K F S H W O R L D
W O P N A V Q X W A A G
O I E O H F H T E N T W
R C E W E E S V F C N Z
D E C L A R E P G H K U
S I H E V R N R L A J W
B R I D E G R O O M K O
U H W G N W O C R P D P
S K I E S Y D L Y I M O
B K O J S V F A Y O Q K
O P W K Z J U I Y N V K
U D I R W A R M T H T L

Psalm 19:1-6

Q A K S A A Z T C V Q M
W P S R O D X E R V X L
L A R H G U I D E S O J
Y B T E E O L J S H C N
C D F E P P O E W Q B O
S O N N R A H D P S N K
L V M V O S R E N K A J
H A G F E T S E R E S D
F L C R O U H T F D S Q
Q L F K W R Z I A O X S
I E X B Y E T E N F C G
R Y W U J S L L N G F X

Psalm 23

Answers: Puzzles pages 19-25

```
P X C E K E V Q X P D H
U B L E S S I N G E P X
R A E M T E N N H U N U
E S A O A A D S K O X E
K A N U N S I D I C L K
B S R N D L C T H R Z Y
V C I T B O A E M D A J
I F C A H R T H N W J Y
T M T I E D I L Q D G Y
N S L N I S O P V V H E
E M E F O U N D E D I B
R G Q O W R Z E Y D N U
```

Psalm 24:1-6

```
Q Q O P M E O S V S S W
D J T R U T H E S D S E
E Y E B W T P Q X U A T
X P J G A A T M O V V Y
B G N P U E Y R W A I Y
L E N E M I E S U X O S
G T E A C H O P E S R F
V U H W C O C Y Q H T V
G S I A P Z C J G O P H
Z O E D W R J U J W G Y
R R E M E M B E R V S O
T X S M B X L G S H U U
```

Psalm 25:1-6

```
O F P X B M K J M M C R
X K M G L O A T F Y U O
H H P O B M W W P E M U
X E N D R E W X N K S D
C L H C O N G O T U P D
E P V A U T I M A F A T
X R L L G B B N H I R D
A A I L H T R G G E E I
L I F E T I M E M L D T
T S T D E L G I A H D V
W E E P I N G E U L I Z
D S S D E P T H S O P M W
```

Psalm 30:1-5

```
A V O Q F V T A Y F J Q
N T R J G U O F A C E S
S R E Z E D G F J O D L
W O A G E E E L S X A A
E U N L C L T I A U O J
R B G O P I H C V S U N
E L E R J V E T E L S E
D E L I V E R E D E L X
Z S I F N R A D I A N T
D R P Y A S O U G H T O
Y M S E N D N T O B W L
B H H T C K Y Y Y Y H P S
```

Psalm 34:1-7

Answers: Puzzles pages 27-33

Psalm 37:3-9

Psalm 46:1-6

Psalm 51:10-15

Psalm 57:7-11

Answers: Puzzles pages 35-41

Psalm 66:1-7

Psalm 86:5-10

Psalm 91:1-5

Psalm 95:1-6

Answers: Puzzles pages 43-49

```
P R O C E S S I O N B F
Z N U D H U A M Q C F K
Y P D E J C D T I J O B
L S X N U C O O M G R U
J O I G Q E N D U R E S
O F H O U S E A S A V E
F K I M H S K Y L N E X
E O J G S O F D O T R J
L M U E Y U R P J M A M
Y O L I G H T N H B V R
B B V S P D Y H S T G M
D Q A E Q P F G A K K O
```

Psalm 118:24-29

```
S A R E V N E F N L E H
Q A C D V D W N G R T E
L H N D Q P X F O I L L
S Y U M Y O S M I G S P
V B W D P K R T N H U R
M Y P Q W E R I G T N C
J I J N V E M W F H F L
A N O E B O S I K A O H
A O R M C E L H V N O W
M O U N T A I N S D T Q
F L H K E E P J J F M H
S H A D E K B R D V E E
```

Psalm 121

```
L F I L L E D D U G M G
A O C D V T E Y N X P P
U R C A R R Y I N G E F
G T C I O E P G M Q T E
H U S T R E A M S M X I
T N S E E D M M R O A J
E E E W Z I O N E A W W
R S A G Q R N H A D T P
B F V R E F G D P O F A
E V E L S V Z P U M H N
Q T M A T W A R O T A H
I B O F I R W O T C J A
```

Psalm 126

```
H Y R D M E C M L I F U
N T D A C W K C P Y O G
B F Q N F B Y R R K N Z
E V A C E S A O A O S T
D E L I G H T W S Z Q M
M M O N T C W N S O A J
I U R G I H Y S E F E H
H S D V M N F A M J R U
O I R W B V G U B Z O M
N C L A R B E G L A D B
O A O V E C U Q Y G M L
R K B L L L C O Z B E E
```

Psalm 149:1-5

Answers: Puzzles pages 51-57

```
Y S M U G H C W U I Y W
S P T B R E A T H G C H
G O R B O Y B R N H Y A
R W U Y S U P I P E M L
E E M N U L S C Y V B T
A R P Z D S V T L W A N
T Q E X A I H G D A L R
N O T P F G N P J P S O
E P R A I S E G O D E H
S U H M T W P W V R Q F
S A N C T U A R Y X Q X
T E A S E Z N L G W J T
```

Psalm 150

```
K A N N P S K S B T T F
B X Z M W E Z X A M P B
C H E H P M M K M V R D
N F N O L P G R A C E N
Y S H I N I N G Z S C D
W R E T C H E F I S I N
B S P C I M K M N H O N
R P H O U N O T G I U B
I E N D U R E S T E S D
G N A G P E E R S L Q C
H B E V W K O S P D J W
T B C S Q P L O I B M M
```

Amazing Grace

```
U C P H Y G S V B F M U
G R K Q R T R I N I T Y
L O V E N O N O H R F G
V W L I T E T P V F F H
X N A D H C A F M Y A U
T S Z M E R C I F U L K
G V Z F E N B N M U L H
I X R S P U E J I F I Y
Y E M O R N I N G U N M
P O W E R P Z U H M G D
Q S H M N Z N H T U O T
A C K T Q H O L Y G C A
```

Holy Holy Holy

```
W O V E R F L O W S A S
K C Q X E A L M W N I U
C A L C F I W N O Y R P
E G P E U T F I R M D P
O L O L G H T P D R E L
Y B F L E A S O K R L Y
M U A E D C W T W A A V
W I X N A P V E C W I F
R V U T R R N N H U D D
K O T L O K N T Y H Q W
F I K J B W A O F B Z C
Z U Y K T P P F T Y G D
```

How Firm a Foundation

108

Answers: Puzzles pages 59-65

Come Thou Fount of Every Blessing

It Is Well

Praise to the Lord the Almighty

Be Thou My Vision

Answers: Puzzles pages 67-73

All Creatures of Our God and King

All Hail the Power of Jesus' Name

To God Be the Glory

In the Sweet By-and-By

Answers: Puzzles pages 75-81

What A Friend We Have in Jesus

His Eye Is on the Sparrow

Battle Hymn of the Republic

Come, Let Us All Go Down

Answers: Puzzles pages 83-89

GHHPDUAZHARY
WYNWOMHWSGAY
LPKFGVBOARHY
LACOLAFRPRLS
HMGRHOTSIUNA
IJMEYAWHFGTI
PLFVNSPIEMHN
RIVERUTPNRRT
KFARIURAYGOS
UOESANGELGNF
CBGEJZGOLDEN
TLBGTKSSSFBD

*Shall We Gather at
the River*

YANNWJUIOXQI
EBBSOCCAAAACC
OKCIGEMSBFTE
DWORDVSABHAO
UXMXPETFWSOM
VWFCNNXGIOWG
ZCOKETNATJIL
BHRIEIQTHONA
MATELDEUMUGN
DASAHELPERSC
PREYLACHANGE
UHAFEEBSAASR

Abide With Me

AWONDROUSBLE
EZXBZEUUYIDM
TTWVLJOYFULL
JHWKEEPJJWXT
HEARTESSHOXL
COUNTLESSRGW
EVUGKCTXELRL
DOQIIFCHUDFC
BIEOIITAOYFL
LCJGQOJNVAGO
GENNMTTDLZCI
RSRNARMSNHXR

*Now Thank We All
Our God*

PACROWNNDKYG
LHRSYNMMMMUL
PQIBCEFEUYJV
OIMATCHLESSA
RASSNEETTTIJ
LNODLBABEIBC
ITNHMNVHRCQZ
KHTDRAECNWBL
HEKADKNGIXAT
BMCMAQLYTYSB
TNGWJTYAYYCD
ICAMNSLXWQTZ

*Crown Him with
Many Crowns*

112

Answers: Puzzles pages 91-97

If You Will Only Let God Guide You

Blessed Assurance

When We Survey the Wondrous Cross

Jesus Paid It All

Answers: Puzzles pages 99-101

I E G E X T F B R G X T
M G B N B A R N N G P K
E B F D S U E I V G G E
M T O U V T L A U J I M
C W R R A I L W S M G I
R P T E A Z D H A O P G
A X R V M C W E N R U H
F H E W X B C L C T K T
T R S K O N L P I A C Y
P Z S M I R I E E L Q X
O R A R M E D R N P K Z
X O P O U Q Z D T O K V

A Mighty Fortress Is Our God

D P H I S H P M A K E R
M E E E I G X Z T R F Z
C C V J G M M H U O C Q
H E V O H Y G T Z K C J
R C W B T I A P S B Y G
I R O L L E D E I I H N
S O V E R E I G N Z V R
T S D C R R E B R F H S
H S S C O D E D V H I L
N F A L A S L M Q N W O
E S G E Z N L J W A I T
U O H W N T F F C Y L Z

At the Cross